RAISING A HIGHLY SENSITIVE CHILD

The Ultimate Guide for Parents of Highly Sensitive Children. Understand Them Better, and Raise Good, Happy, and Emotionally Intelligent Kids

ALISSA TAYLOR

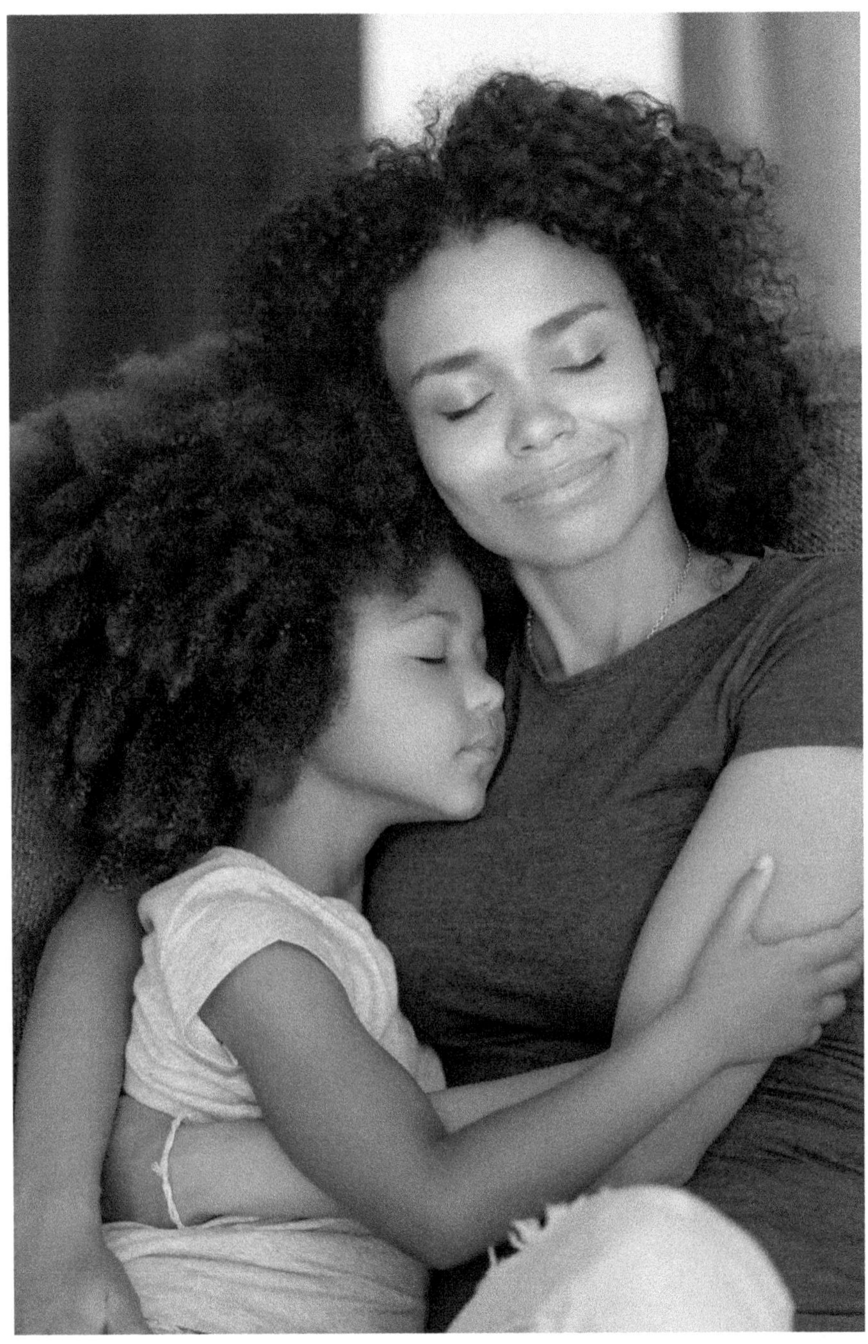

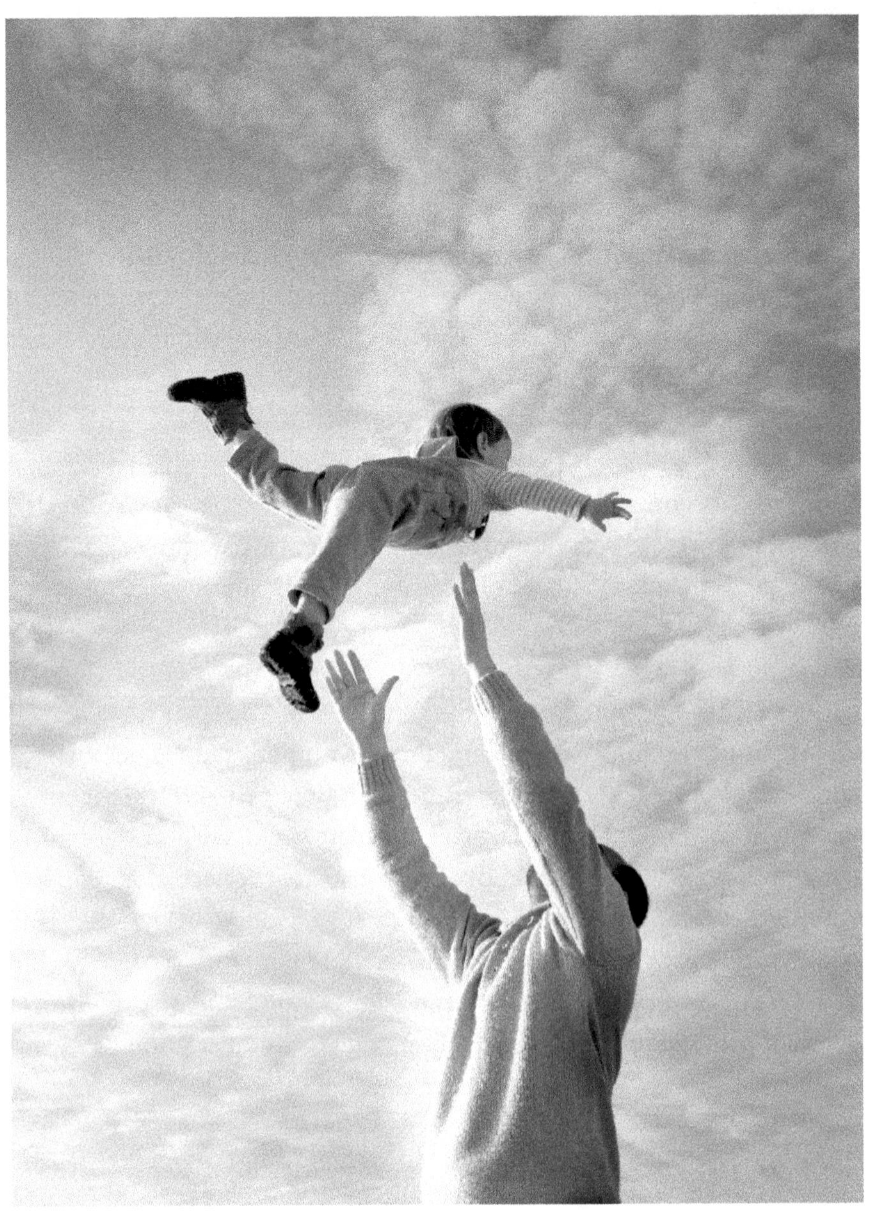

Table of Content

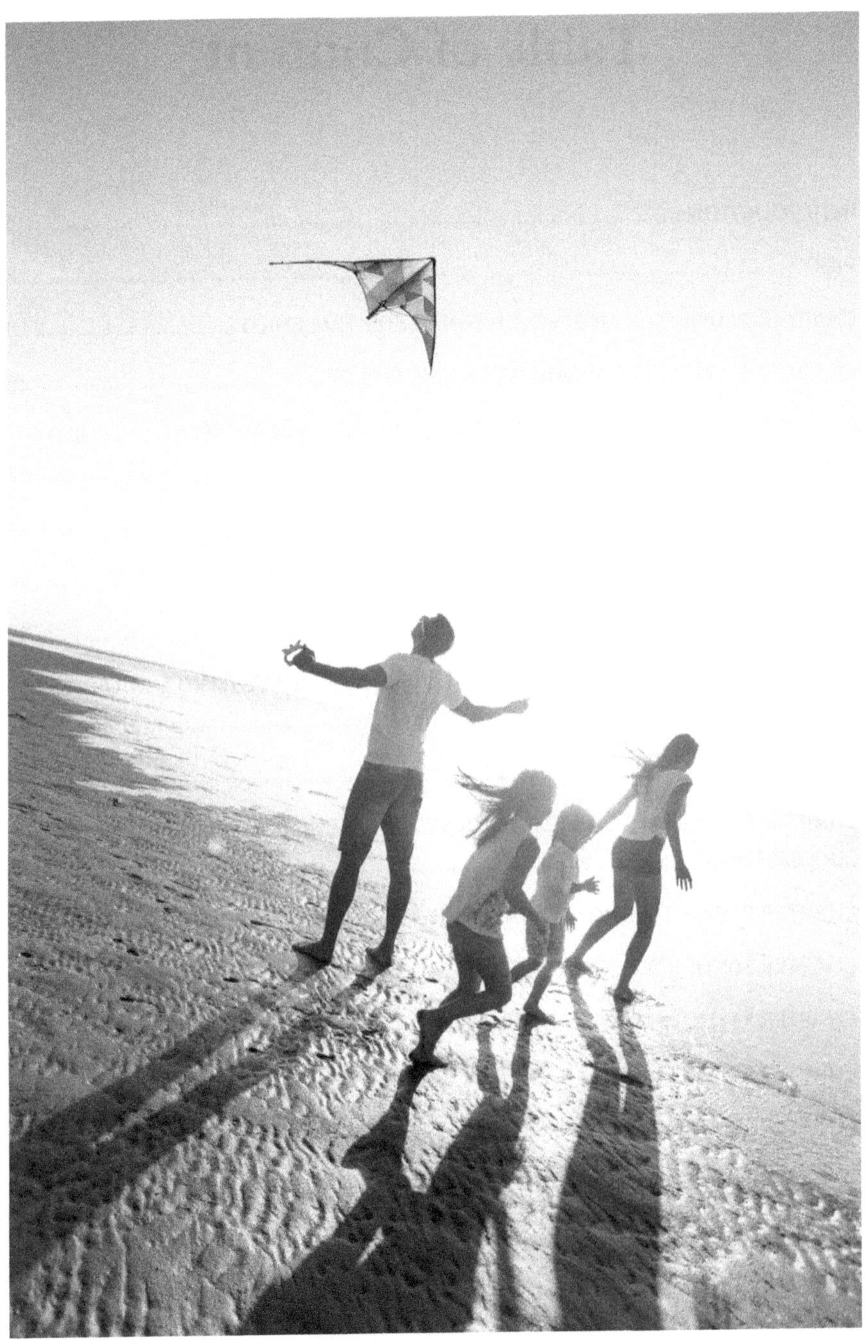

Introduction

Many children are born with heightened sensitivity to their environment, and they will need a lot of patience, understanding, and acceptance as they learn about themselves and their world. It can be tempting as parents to want them to be more like our other children, who seem relatively easygoing, but we cannot get frustrated when we see that our sensitivity no longer needs the same attention that he did before.

What we need to do is focus instead on building up this child's self-esteem, so he or she doesn't feel like he or she needs to "do anything" in order for others to notice him or her. The most important thing we need to know is that we simply cannot change a highly sensitive child. We can try to help them learn ways of calming themselves, so they feel less overwhelmed by their sensitivities, but it will never be possible for them to be the same as other children. Instead, we must praise them for their special traits and work with them on developing skills to deal with the world, one at a time. It can get very difficult when you are dealing with a sensitive child who doesn't seem to want your help and just wants you to leave him or her alone.

As the parent of a sensitive child, you will need to learn to have a lot of patience and to be very observant. Sensitive children are often showing major signs of distress, but they may not be able to verbalize what is bothering them. Their strong emotions can also get in the way of them wanting to seek help from you, so you may need to sit down and work with them so they can learn some self-regulation skills. As a mom with a highly sensitive child myself, I know how difficult it can be when your child desires more attention than you feel comfortable giving.

I recommend that you listen to your child's needs and try to meet them in whatever way you can, rather than trying to change their behavior. We may find comfort in trying to teach our children ways of ignoring fears or controlling their feelings, but we must always make sure that we don't ignore the basic needs of our sensitive child. As time went by, it turned into the joy of being able to create an ideal family environment for the child's growth. Most parents have a misconception about the highly sensitive child. They think that this is a child who is "too sensitive." This could not be further from the truth.

Children with this sensitivity are very perceptive, and they can foresee things that we never imagined. This may scare many people, especially when they see how much this child cares about others and how far he or she will go to help them. The thing we need to remember is that all children are born with different personalities, and it would be impossible for us to change a highly sensitive child into someone else. It is best to adapt our child's personality to his or her own strengths and weaknesses and focus on what needs love. When it comes to raising a highly sensitive child, we cannot try to change them into something they are not. Emotionally charged children will need their parents and us to become more attuned and compassionate toward them. We need strong support from our spouses so we can be there when we need them in the best way possible. It is very important for us to know that there are many resources for people with ADHD, as well as depression, anxiety disorders, Asperger's syndrome, etc.

For example, children with Asperger's syndrome are sometimes sensitive to sound and other elements of the environment. So it is essential for us as parents to be very observant in order to know exactly what might be bothering them. This will allow us to act and respond immediately and try to offer solutions before the problem gets too big.

PART I

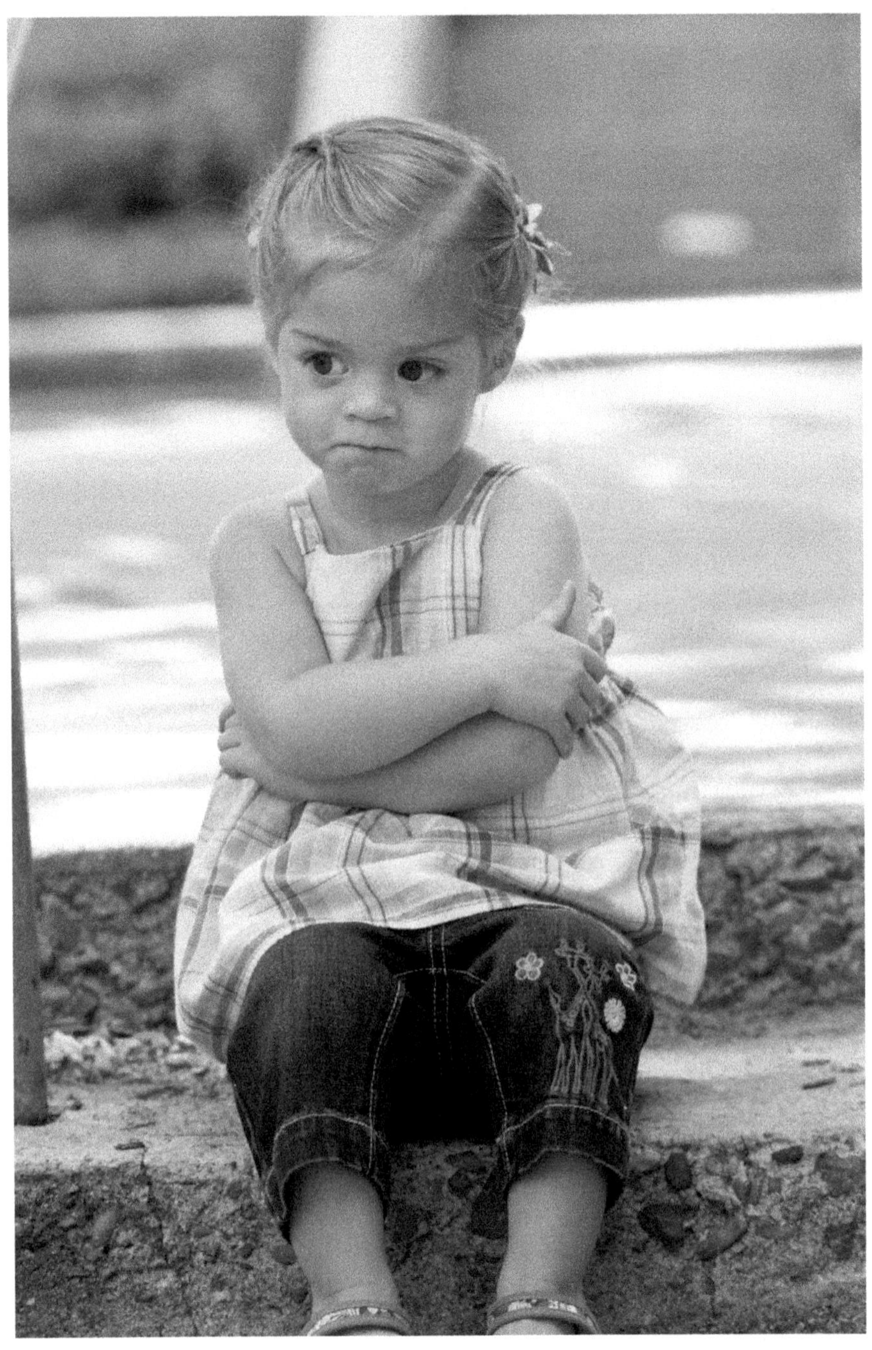

CHAPTER 1:

Understanding a Highly Sensitive Child

Highly sensitive kids become overwhelmed easily. They often cry, worry about getting into trouble frequently, and require a great deal of reassurance. They also feel every emotion intensely. That means they're likely to become overexcited, extra angry, and super scared. Even when it comes to everyday events, emotionally sensitive children are usually very tuned into their feelings. They take things personally, and they don't forget a slight. Here's a list of "high sensitivity traits" that both my book and research have identified. Think of them as clues that your child might be emotionally sensitive:

In addition to this list of traits, there are certain behaviors that can clue you into whether your child is high in sensitivity: crying easily, worrying a lot, being easily hurt by teasing or criticism, engaging in "catastrophizing," feeling guilty without cause, discussing their problems with friends often or wishing they were better off than they are. You may also notice that some of the high-sensitivity behaviors listed above have been linked to some of the common symptoms of autism spectrum disorder (ASD). These include extreme sensitivity to sensory input, difficulty with social interaction, and obsessive behaviors. High sensitivity is a trait that runs in families. While it's not always present in a child who has ASD, when it is present, it's very likely that he or she has ASD. About 10% of all children are developmentally normal despite being very sensitive and easily overwhelmed by their surroundings and emotions. Those with high sensitivity tend to do better academically, socially, and in emotionally demanding careers.

1. Emotionally sensitive kids are very emotional and often despair of ever being happy again. They cling to their parents or are extremely dependent on them. These kids are more likely to hurt themselves or set themselves on fire without realizing it. They're also likely to try too hard sometimes when

they should just chill out. When they're upset with a friend, they'll keep texting and calling until their friend talks to them again or gives them a callback.

2. They're very sensitive to criticism and will take things personally, even when they shouldn't. Even a small remark about how they're doing something "wrong" will be enough to hurt their feelings. These kids are also likely to worry a lot about what others think of them. This is one of the behaviors that is commonly associated with autism spectrum disorder (ASD), but it's not always present in those who have ASD.
3. They're also easily hurt by teasing or criticism, which may cause them to be less sociable or shy than other kids their age. In fact, they may find it hard just being around other people unless they know them well and trust that they have good intentions.
4. They take things very personally, even when they shouldn't. Even a slight from someone they love will cause these kids to feel upset for days on end.
5. They worry about their problems excessively and don't know how to solve them. They're likely to ask you questions about their problems until you can give them a good solution or until they feel better about it somehow. In some cases, these kids may have repetitive behaviors that serve as something of a "solution" to their problems (such as rocking back and forth in order to calm down). In other cases, however, they just worry about their problems until they can come up with a solution by themselves or with your help.
6. They're often (very) hyperaware of their own personal safety and the safety of those around them. They may be overly cautious about things like falling, fire alarms, germs, or other threats to their well-being. They also tend to be more easily scared than other kids and are likely to avoid situations that might cause them to fear.
7. They have a hard time making friends without special help, and they can't seem to tune out an argument. However, when they do make friends, they tend to have very loyal ones because they don't want to lose their closest friends over something silly or because they're annoyed by someone else behaving badly toward them.

8. They don't believe they're in trouble until it's too late. They may be late for school, work, or a play or other activity, but it'll only dawn on them once they're trapped in a hairy situation, and the teacher starts calling their name.
9. They can take things very personally when others are angry at them and may become enraged about it. This causes them to negatively judge other people, which can end up in them saying mean things about other people out of anger and frustration. Others may hurt their feelings by teasing or simply not acting nice to them as others would expect. These kids may become very emotional when they feel others aren't treating them fairly or with respect. As a result, they're likely to cry easily when they're hurt.
10. They can be obsessed with fixing the problems that have been troubling them. They'll do anything to make sure they never have to face that problem again and that it stays away from their family and friends too.
11. They have a hard time relaxing and making the most of situations that should be fun for them, even though they really want to enjoy themselves in these situations. They may have a hard time just being themselves, and they might not want to do anything simply for fun or because it's interesting.
12. They can take things really seriously and can become overly distressed about them, even when they should think the situation isn't that serious. This can cause them to hide their feelings from others or pretend that everything is fine so everyone doesn't worry about them. They may also try to hide the fact that they're hurt by not talking about it or pretending that something minor happened instead of dealing with the actual problem. Unfortunately, no one learns from pretending they would rather deal with problems sooner than later (and if we're honest, pretending is what helped us avoid some situations in the first place).
13. They feel defeated by small problems and can't think of ways to solve them by themselves. Of course, if they can't solve the problem by themselves, they may become overwhelmed with self-doubt and a lack of confidence. They might even start to believe that their problems are so great that there's no one else who can help them solve them, which is very untrue.

14. Their lives are almost always hectic because their mind is one big jumble of thoughts that get stuck in loops over and over again (i.e., stuck in a habitual way). They may also feel very anxious even when it doesn't make sense for them too because their anxiety has become so habitual as well.
15. They have a hard time getting into other people's minds and feel disconnected from everyone because their mind just goes off at random. These children trust their feelings more than the inner voice inside of their own head, which at times can lead to them becoming very frustrated when they can't understand what someone is thinking or why they're acting differently than they should be.
16. They think that things will never get better for them, even when they're doing well in school and making friends, but these kids have a hard time believing that they'll make any progress in life as well when change doesn't occur right away. They are always thinking about the "big picture" and don't seem to be able to appreciate the small good things that happen throughout the day.
17. They have a hard time paying attention in class because their thoughts are everywhere else but where they should be. They may even have a hard time understanding what someone is saying or asking them to do because they're always having to explain things over and over again.
18. Nothing seems to motivate these children anymore, not even rewards or incentives (i.e., "carrots on a stick"). They will work hard to get the things they want because they believe that doing so will solve all their problems and make them feel better, but it doesn't. Things don't change with these children because they don't change at all.
19. They don't want to be seen as the victim and think that everybody else is at fault for not understanding them or making their life easier for them by just listening. In other words, well-meaning people can become just as frustrating as their parents when dealing with these kids because trying to counsel them and talk things out with them sometimes doesn't work either.

20. They have a hard time recognizing the love within others and are extremely mistrusting everyone. This is often because they have had people try to help them, with no results.
21. They never feel like they have enough of anything for themselves and need to control others in order to get what they want.
22. They're extremely afraid of everything from being abandoned, to controlled, to having things taken away from them and are vigilant about it. This causes them issues with trust, intimacy, and even their own happiness because so much revolves around not trusting that if something goes wrong, it will be the end of their world. It never occurs the other way around where their world will only go on if things go right.
23. They have a hard time trusting anyone they don't know too well, and even then, they may wonder if that person is really trustworthy for good or if they're hiding something from them.
24. They have a hard time knowing when to stop talking, which can make others think they're controlling, bossy, and even annoying. This is because their mind moves so quickly from one thought to the next that they're not able to stop when someone else would be able to easily understand that the conversation may need to end soon. Other times these kids are simply nervous when speaking in front of other people or in new situations and just don't know how to act their age.
25. They feel extremely sorry for themselves and think that there's no place in the world for them. Everything is hard for them to handle, and they don't want to put forth any effort into doing the simplest of things because they can't stand dealing with the inevitable problems it will cause them.
26. They have difficulty making friends because they're shy and don't trust easily until they know that someone can be trusted. If that happens, these kids can become very loyal friends who will always have someone there to talk to about their problems, no matter how trivial and embarrassing they may seem to be to others.
27. Their listening skills are very poor because their mind is always on the go, and they are often drifting off into a daydream when someone else is talking. They may not be able to focus on a

subject going on right in front of their face because they keep glancing over at something else that catches their eye.

28. They're very forgetful about things like remembering what they did yesterday, where they're going, or how to do something. These kids have a hard time storing things in the first place because it's just too much information for them to process and store properly in their brains. Another reason they have a hard time remembering things is that their mind just doesn't stay on one topic long enough to make sense of it and force it into memory.
29. They don't understand why they can't do things others claim are so simple (although this doesn't mean they're not smart), especially when others can do it easily for them and even if they don't understand it themselves or how to do it something.
30. They are very sensitive to things and become very upset when they are perceived as being wrong or treated in a way that doesn't make them feel respected. This is because their mind is so full of thoughts or fears that they're not able to process what would be considered "normal" behavior (i.e., thoughts are "off the wall").
31. They don't trust anyone, especially people who are established (i.e., "old"). Even when they're trying to talk to and trust people, these kids are suspicious of them, which causes them not to give others the benefit of the doubt if only for their own safety.
32. They have a hard time trusting that things will turn out all right because even though some things may look good on the outside, their mind can still be playing tricks on them and causing them to worry about things that aren't really a problem.
33. They feel like their parents, or other adults are making them do everything, even when they don't want to. They also believe that this is why other kids hate them because they're always being told what to do and may be treated differently than others as a result of it.
34. They have a hard time knowing when to stop talking or stop worrying about something, which can cause them more stress in the long run, although they don't realize this because the stress will build on itself after a while if not relieved through

telling someone else or by doing something that makes them feel better (e.g., exercising).

35. They are very insecure about themselves because just as they feel like things will never get better in their life, they also feel like they'll never have a good life. They are always worrying about the future and can't enjoy life or what's happening at present because of these negative feelings.
36. They may have an overall sense of being different and not fitting in with anyone else. They may think that everyone else is mad at them or thinks that something is wrong with them. They may even think that others want to hurt them out of jealousy or because they're envious of all the problems these kids have, although the truth might be that nobody around them understands what it's really like for these children and what it feels like being them.
37. They try to hide how they're feeling with the age-old trick of pretending everything is fine even when they're not. They can also be very good at "saving face" with other people by pretending things are fine, although they know inside that they're actually pretty upset and hurting in a lot of different ways that make them very uncomfortable near others.
38. They care too much about what other people think or say or do or how things turn out for them, so bad things happen because of this. They also care too much about themselves, which causes them to have low self-esteem, poor body image, and feel overly sorry for themselves.
39. They let the small things get to them and can't seem to enjoy anything anymore because they're always looking for things that will make them happy, but nothing ever does.
40. They are extremely moody and emotional because their ability to reason with their own feelings is stunted or non-existent. They can also have a hard time behaving appropriately when they feel this way, which is why many of these children end up being labeled as troublemakers or bad influences on other kids.
41. They have a hard time sleeping because their mind keeps moving every time they close their eyes, and they also get very tense when they're trying to fall asleep. This causes them to stay up later than most, and because they've been so restless all

day, it also makes it difficult for them to get a good night's sleep.

42. They have a hard time concentrating and can't seem to focus or think about anything other than what's bothering them in the moment, which is usually what's going wrong with their life at that particular point in time in the first place (this is because there are too many thoughts going through their mind from so many different angles).
43. They have a hard time making decisions and feel in control of their life. They'll feel like they can do anything in the world, but nothing will ever turn out right for them, which is partly because they feel that their mind is so confused that nothing is coming to them easily anymore.
44. They have a hard time forming relationships with other people because their mind is too scattered and busy to focus on anything other than isolating themselves from everyone else, including what's going on around them at the moment, and focusing more on the things that worry them (i.e., they're just not able to get comfortable with where they are) or what keeps bothering them in the first place (i.e., they're not able to get comfortable with themselves).
45. They have a hard time making decisions because they often won't know what they want or need and yet will think that they are fully capable of getting it. Sometimes their mind can be so focused on one thing that it makes it so they don't even know what else is going on in the world at the moment that would make them happy, but even if all this is true for other people, there will still be times when these kids will not know what to do with themselves because their mind has no idea.
46. They think that people can tell when they're making faces or that other people can read their minds, which causes them to be afraid of everything and everyone. They also don't trust other people because they don't think anyone will ever really know what is going on with them (which may actually be true), so it's to the point where they're not even sure if they want to make any effort to get to know others in the first place, and if so what those relationships should be like.
47. They have a hard time recognizing when things are wrong for them or that there's even anything wrong in the first place.

They can have difficulty knowing what to do if something is wrong, and even when they do know it's wrong for them, they can't handle the consequences that go along with being in the wrong.

48. They are extremely cautious about getting into relationships because they don't want to be hurt, and their mind might even tell them that other people are going to hurt or abandon them. The truth is that most people get into relationships hoping that things won't end up giving either one of them pain, which means that these kids may not be wholly correct in their fears and need to let themselves get used to the idea that they'll need to move out of their comfort zone a bit.
49. They have a hard time trusting other people or their own instincts. Sometimes these kids' minds will tell them that they can't trust anyone, but when they've learned that this isn't true, it may also cause them to have a hard time knowing who they do trust and when they can trust someone else.
50. They have a hard time feeling in control of their thoughts because most of the time, these kids feel like it's impossible for them to do anything right (i.e., a lot of things are simply "off the wall" for them). They also have a hard time telling how someone else is feeling because they're so caught up in their own head that there's no way to know what's going on.
51. If they see something out of the ordinary or someone does something out-of-character, it makes them extremely uncomfortable, and they may even become overly defensive because they'll just feel like someone has hurt them in some way from nothing at all, even though this isn't the case. They do this because their mind is so focused on what is wrong with their life that anything that happens to them will automatically be viewed as "wrong" by these children, and thus they'll need to defend themselves against it.
52. They become very secretive because they believe that people talk about them behind their back, and so, therefore, there's no point in telling anyone what they're thinking or feeling because everyone will just feel sorry for them and not really care.
53. They tend to think that other people are ESP or mind-readers who can tell what's going on with them even when it's not true at all, which causes beyond-their-control paranoia. This is

particularly true with other kids who will tease these children cruelly because of this (i.e., "you're getting married!" "No, I'm not," "yes, you are!").

54. They can't have any meaningful relationships with anyone because the person they feel most comfortable with is themselves, and the only one they trust is their mind (which, again, can be more trouble than help sometimes).
55. They are very picky about what they eat or drink and can't stand to have other people tell them what to do or when they should do something else instead. They also don't like to be told that something doesn't have to go a certain way.
56. They get very agitated or upset if someone tries to help them with something because they can't understand why anyone would do this and can't believe that people want to be so nice and kind to them. They often won't want to accept the help because it makes them feel like they're a burden on people, even though this is not their intention at all.
57. They don't like to be told what to do, which is because their mind just doesn't know how to process these types of orders, but they also don't like when things go wrong for them or when other people do more work for them.
58. They can't understand why they're still alive sometimes because the mind is so focused on death and dying that it makes it hard for these individuals to have a good grasp of what's going on in their life. They will often feel like everything is happening to them against their will or that they would be better off dead because nothing will ever turn out for them, so the harder someone else tries to make things work for them, the more that person may feel like they've failed or made a mistake in doing so, even though this isn't necessarily true at all.
59. They have a hard time with being in relationships because they can't slow down their mind and just be with the person they're with right now. They will think that other people are going to break them and that things are better alone, even though this is not true at all.
60. They have a hard time accepting gifts and treats from others because their mind just doesn't know how to deal with these sorts of things, so it says that nothing ever pleased them before (usually this is true), but the truth is that these children want to

please people because they don't want to make anyone feel bad or make them think badly about themselves.

61. They feel overly nervous or insecure a lot of the time and can't always tell why these feelings are there, which causes them to think that the world is against them.
62. They have a hard time doing things at the moment and need to prepare for everything first before anything else happens in their day or at any other time (i.e., they must do all their work before they can go outside and play because that's what makes them happy).
63. They have a hard time doing things at the moment because they just can't get their mind to stop thinking about what will happen next or what they're going to need or want in the future, which makes everything seem like work and causes them to be on-edge and unfocused.
64. They have a hard time doing things at the moment because they don't know how they'll feel about something, and so there's no point in them actually doing it (something that, again, never bothered anyone else before).
65. They have a hard time understanding how to make other people happy because their mind is too scattered and busy for this to be any kind of reality for these children.
66. They have a hard time sleeping because they're always thinking of something else to do and are likely worrying about something that may happen or because of the occurrences that just occurred. This can also cause them to have a hard time falling asleep because they can't relax.
67. They have a hard time stopping their mind from thinking about things, which causes them to be very hard on themselves when they just don't know what is going on with themselves anymore and simply want to stop thinking about it all for a while.
68. They are highly self-critical and can't believe what everyone else thinks of them because they're so focused on their own faults and failures that they don't know what to make of it all.
69. They feel as though they're being taken advantage of by others because their mind is too scattered to be able to tell anyone what's truly going on with them or even if there's any point for

other people helping them out (i.e., "why would anyone want to help me?").

70. They have a hard time dealing with problems because their mind just doesn't know how to be reasonable about things anymore. This can cause them to over-think things or over-complicate everything, even though things in the years before were simple for them as well.
71. They are always concerned about the future and feel like they won't have enough money or that they'll live a life of poverty and struggle, which is why they're always trying to plan ahead for everything or trying to figure out what's going on in their head so that they can make the right choice.
72. They are self-conscious about their appearance because they can't stop thinking about how they look, which is why they'll try and take care of themselves so that no one knows how bad off they really are. They don't want to be seen as unattractive or disgusting to others, but instead as someone who is weak (and thus not worth caring for), which is why it's to the point where their appearance matters more than others do (i.e., "what exactly am I supposed to look like?").
73. They often have a hard time connecting emotionally with others because they're too busy feeling sorry for themselves and living in the past or future, which makes them seem distant or disconnected from almost everyone.
74. They can't seem to focus on what people are saying because their mind is in a million places all at once and so they tend to just stare at people and not get anything positive out of it.
75. They can't seem to be happy because they live in fear of everything and everyone, which causes them to have a hard time getting anything else other than work out right for them.
76. They always want something to go right for them, even if it's something small or irrelevant, but most of the time, this is preventing them from actually enjoying things in life because they're too busy focusing on how all the good things won't be enough for them or what's "wrong" with their life instead (i.e. "it's not enough").
77. They can't enjoy anything because they're always in the wrong, even if they're just doing what someone else wants them to do.

They also can't seem to understand how something could make them happy because their mind is too preoccupied.

78. They feel like they're being forced into things because their mind won't let them think otherwise and feel like everyone else is judging them for it (when no one ever cared about this in the first place).
79. They have a hard time with anger because of the overthinking and fear that their mind is constantly creating for them, which causes them to only be upset when they feel like they've done something wrong and not for any reason at all.
80. They have a hard time being playful because their mind is so focused on all the things they worry about that they don't leave any room for fun. This can cause them to just feel "uptight" and stressed out instead of like themselves at all, which isn't healthy to begin with, but it becomes even worse when it's caused by something as simple as trying to have fun.
81. They can't always tell what's going on in someone else's head and are very self-critical because of this, even though they would've had no trouble understanding another person before.
82. They have a hard time seeing the people around them as real people because they feel like they're not normal people like themselves or that others aren't actually as good as they are.
83. They often feel like everyone is against them and against their family, which causes them to feel panicked that people will just harm their family members (which has never proven true before).
84. They often feel like they have no control over their thoughts or emotions, which sometimes causes them to act out because they're simply not comfortable with what's going on inside of them at all.
85. They always want people to know that they can't be put down or let out, and, in fact, they will fight back against any sort of negativity that is headed toward them.
86. They focus on things outside themselves and don't really care about the way other people are feeling because what can they do about it? The negative thoughts inside their head are distracting enough for them without having to think about others (i.e., "why are you crying?" "Because something happened").

87. They have a hard time understanding how to help someone because their mind is too preoccupied with what's going on inside of them to even consider that they might be able to help someone else.
88. They are very emotional and sensitive, but not in a way that makes them seem like they're overly emotional; instead, it just causes them to take things personally when they're not at all.
89. Their minds are always going and working overtime, but again this isn't something that seems like a positive thing for other people (i.e., "how can you think so fast?!").
90. They think of all the things that can go wrong and how everything will never work out for them, which causes them to have a hard time getting anything to go right for themselves.
91. They feel like there is no reason for people to be nice to them or other people in general (i.e., why should anyone treat me well if I can't treat myself well?).
92. They feel like their life is meaningless because they don't know how to find purpose in their lives anymore, which is why it doesn't matter if they do something else that they enjoy or if they make friends with someone else—it won't make a difference either way.
93. They have a hard time trusting people because they're too scared to make mistakes that will tell everyone all of their secrets and cause problems for them in the future, which is why they don't tell anyone anything (i.e., "why should I trust you?" "I don't know you well enough").
94. They are very self-critical because their minds are so overworked and distracted that they can't be relied upon to do their part, which is why it's hard for others to depend on them (i.e., "you're not taking this seriously enough").
95. They have a hard time understanding relationships between people, especially romantic ones.
96. They have a hard time accepting compliments, gifts, or treats from others because their mind suddenly believes that everyone is looking evil and trying to hurt them (which has never happened before).
97. They can't understand what would make anyone like them because their minds are too scattered and full of negative thoughts for this to be true for any of these children.

98. They feel as though they have no friends because their mind is so full of fear that they just don't know how to interact with other people, which means that they're alone by default (i.e., "why would anyone like me?" "I'm not likable").
99. They feel like they've always been a bad person because of all the things that have gone wrong for them and how they've been treated by others, which makes them feel like a loser and unlikable.
100. They feel as though their lives are meaningless and can't understand why everyone is ignoring their existence—it just doesn't matter to anyone what happened to them or what's going on with them inside of their head.

CHAPTER 2:

What is a Highly Sensitive Child?

The scientific name is sensory processing sensitivity. It's not a disease, nor does it develop over time. It's temperament, and about one in five kids is born with it. A High Sensitivity Child is one who "feels deeply" and "takes in the world around them." HSCs have a higher need for order, routine, and predictability. The typical child has a threshold of about 20 minutes before they're overstimulated and upset. A High-Sensitive Child may only take five minutes before they are crying or freaking out because it's just too much. It's not that these kids cannot calm down or don't feel loved—it's that they are overwhelmed with stimuli. They also have high levels of empathy but a lower ability to be assertive, persistent, or independent. They tend to be creative, curious, and idealistic. They are often introverted and have a rich inner life. And they may struggle with sensory-overload issues, processing speed, perfectionism, depression, or anxiety.

Highly Sensitive Children (HSCs) are different from other kids in their nervous system's responses to stimuli. They actually have a low threshold for stimulation—they feel things more intensely than others do. HSCs are more easily overwhelmed, but the flip side is that they're also more deeply affected by beauty and deeply moved by emotion. Children with sensory-processing differences also process information more slowly than most children. They are often perfectionists because their brains work slowly, taking in all the information they can before deciding what to do. Their perfectionism comes from wanting to take in all the information possible to make sure there aren't any mistakes. This same trait may also cause a tendency toward anxiety and/or depression. More information is being processed, and when those decisions are made slowly, more feelings of not enough time and less-than can be part of the package.

HSCs love deeply, but they can also have more trouble being assertive or independently persistent. They tend to be creative as well as anxious and sensitive to criticism. They are often introverted, quiet types who draw inside themselves for comfort. They form deep bonds with the people they love, but not without a struggle. Because their nervous systems react so strongly to stimuli, they have a hard time managing their emotions from moment to moment.

Children with sensory processing differences may struggle with sensory-overload issues. These children can be very sensitive to light, sound, touch, taste, and smell. They need time away from the nonstop stimulation of our culture: lots of breaks to run and jump and climb; quiet time alone in their rooms so they can decompress; soft fabrics against their skin to feel more grounded; foods that don't have strong textures or tastes. Children with sensory processing differences often have difficulty managing stress and frustration. They tend to react more strongly than other kids to disappointment, sadness, hunger, or fatigue. Ear-piercing screams of frustration are common for these children because they feel things deeply and have trouble regulating intense emotions.

As adults, HSCs often move away from their families to avoid the overwhelming stimuli of everyday life. They need their own space and quiet time to process information. Like any trait, this is not all bad: they are creative and passionate people who often have deep inner lives. Some become highly successful in music, art, design, or writing. They tend to be empathetic and get deeply involved with causes they care about. With enough support, many do well in school; others struggle with feelings of not being good enough or recognized for their talents. Those who are not given enough support may become perfectionists, shy, or depressed. Some HSCs do well in the classroom but have trouble with emotional outbursts, difficulty staying organized and on task, or being assertive. Some excel in school but find it difficult to make friends because of the way they process information. Most of them deal with a combination of these issues, so it’s important to understand how this can affect them in school and at home.

High Sensitivity Training

The High Sensitivity Training (HST) program was developed by Dr. Elaine Aron using behavioral science research. This program was first used in group therapy sessions but has been proven to be effective for individual therapy as well. The behavioral skills developed for HST include:

1. Sensory Stripping

This is a very simple idea. HSCs tend to think about things in extreme ways. When someone voices an opinion that is different from your own, it can be very uncomfortable. When you hear the tone of the voice, you may react by thinking, "That person is so mean" or "That person is so stupid!" As a result of this reaction, you automatically begin filtering out that person's input from your mind. The idea of Sensory Stripping is to learn how to ignore what you don't like and use the short-term memory to focus on what you do like. Begin by noticing your thoughts about a situation or person, but then strip away the thoughts that are not positive ones. Leave only those that are positive.

2. Energy In

This is a process of cooling off by slowing down and calming your body down. You can also imagine yourself as an ice cube melting in a cup of hot coffee. You can imagine your body as a pool of warm water and then gradually refill that pool with cool water. If someone is yelling at you, you can imagine the words being like a piece of paper blowing by.

3. The Stress/Trauma Trigger Workbook

This workbook helps HSCs understand their body's reaction to stress triggers, how to calm down fast, and how to take care of their body when it needs extra support. It includes many helpful examples for a variety of stress triggers such as hospitals, crowds, crying babies, loud noises, or public speaking. This workbook can be found at http://www.hiyhac.com/library/index.php?cat=1&pub=25&title=The+Stress+Trigger+Workbook

The HST Program is currently being used in Italy, the United Kingdom, and the United States, as well as in other countries.

Individual treatment needs vary for HSCs, given that they often have more than one type of issue and additional needs such as anxiety issues and OCD, and therefore, therapy should be tailored to each individual's needs. As a rule, HSCs tend to receive more aggressive and direct therapies in which they learn new coping skills for reacting to their triggers and social situations. Treatment often starts with a set period of time to adjust to the therapy environment but continues long after that. Some clinics offer more intensive treatment as well. Individual therapy is not always required for HSCs, but it can give them insight into even deeper issues such as what causes them emotional distress and what defensive behaviors they may have incorporated into their daily lives.

They are often very uncertain about the right treatment path. That is one of the main reasons why support is important for HSCs and their clinicians. In time the HSC needs to be able to recognize the difference between situations that are more stressful than usual and those that are more traumatic. This learning may happen in both individual and group therapy sessions.

The therapist may be able to identify the types of triggers that seem to lead to severe tantrums or trigger episodes, the main one being when an HSC has a combination of high expectations about other people's reactions and a feeling of being overwhelmed with competence demands.

They must take responsibility for what is happening in their body during these triggering conditions and learn how to calm themselves down completely. There are several techniques that can be used to help with stress and anxiety levels: HSCs tend to be uncomfortable when their therapist is not in the office. It is helpful if the therapist makes themselves available by phone, email, or text at all times. The HSC always needs to know their therapist is willing to talk at any time and can understand what they may need at a given moment. The HSC will appreciate this greatly.

The HSC feels most comfortable when they have some sense of what other people think about them. The HSC would rather hear positive feedback than negative feedback, but negative feedback is better than no feedback at all. HSCs know that they are a bit different from other people and want to be reassured that their differences are acceptable or even desirable. One of the most important ways that HSCs experience feedback is by observing other people's reactions to themselves. This includes such things as facial expressions, body language, tone of voice, and the like. If they are conscious of something special about themselves (something "different" or "unique"), they want to make sure that others see it too. They may dress in a certain style, adopt an unusual accent, or take on a strange mannerism in order to make sure everyone notices this particular characteristic about themselves—and finds it acceptable and perhaps even admirable. For them, feedback from others about their characteristics is very important. They want to be special, and they need to know that being different is okay.

It's important to remember that HSCs are often uncomfortable in groups and are not always skilled at getting what they need from social situations. It's easy for them to feel overwhelmed or criticized in group situations or even individual situations. As a result, they may not ask for what they need, or if they do ask, they may be unaware of the most effective ways to get people to help them in a way that doesn't make them feel overwhelmed. Individual therapy can help them learn effective ways of getting what they want from others and how to listen, observe, and understand other people's reactions. The workbook helps them with sensory stripping and energy techniques. HSCs need feedback from their therapists to learn how to understand what other people are thinking when they are not direct.

Many practitioners rely on "their own" experience with these gifted children. And some have very limited experience with highly sensitive children. The old adage about apples and oranges is true for most of us regarding sensitivity to stimulation: we know apple tastes good, but we may not recognize the difference between that apple and an orange. Our common cultural bias is that children who are highly sensitive to certain stimuli are just being "spoiled,"; and if there is anything wrong, it's the parents' fault. But if these children's highly tuned nervous systems are not respected and honored, they will behave in ways that will elicit more criticism. They will become anxious and emotional, or they will go on an "auto-pilot" to avoid the intense emotions their experiences evoke. As an individual therapist specializing in sensory processing differences, I have found that keeping records of a child's behaviors over time has proven very helpful in making sense of what may be going on with an HSC/HSP. This record-keeping gives me a timeline of when things happened. I can notice patterns in the life of a child and begin to figure out why they are behaving in certain ways. For example, keeping track of when changes occur: a new baby in the family; moving from an apartment to a house; starting a new school; going to summer camp or away to visit relatives; changing preschools, etc., will allow me to see if there might be connections between these events and the behavior changes I am seeing in the child. Then I can ask what may have been happening at those times that might have been stressful. Some practitioners rely on personality tests. There are many good tests available, but not all of them are appropriate for HSCs/HSPs. A few are: The most widely used sensory sensitivity questionnaire is the Sensory Profile (SP).

This questionnaire is geared toward determining the "average" HSC in an average sample group of children. It does not take into account the individual differences that are part of each child's sensitive nervous system, and that can impact their test scores. The SP is not a reliable way to diagnose or assess for a Sensory Processing Disorder (SPD).

There is no one that fits all the approaches to treating HSCs. There are many different issues that affect them, many of which can be resolved at once or at least reduced in severity. The most important factor throughout the process of therapy for this population is respect for their nervous system and its specific needs. Empathy and understanding will go a long way toward reducing anxiety and improving the quality of life for an HSC.

Sensory processing sensitivity "needs" vary from person to person, but there are some general guidelines:

Dr. Elaine Aron, Ph.D. in her book The Highly Sensitive Person: How to Thrive When the World Overwhelms You, recommends a series of self-help books that are written in plain English for children and adults to use in reading up on the topics of HSP neurobiology, temperament theory, and treatment.

CHAPTER 3:

Some of the Common Traits that Highly Sensitive Child Display

1. Emotional

All kids can be emotional. But what if they are more emotional than other kids? This is one of the traits that highly sensitive children display. Some may say it's a blessing, but many parents say it's a curse.

They have a rich and deep inner life. They have an intense curiosity about things around them, and this can lead to meltdowns when they are overwhelmed by too much going on at once or if something is upsetting to them. Parents who also classify as highly sensitive themselves often find themselves totally consumed with the emotions and reactions of their own children, even before reacting to the situation at hand! This can cause enormous strain on relationships with other family members as well as friends, leading to even more emotional responses in return... and the cycle continues.

These unique children are highly affected by their environments. They can be greatly influenced by the feelings and moods of those around them, especially parents, siblings, classmates, or teachers. They feel things deeply and therefore have a hard time when exposed to things like loud noises or large amounts of chaos around them. A highly sensitive child will tend to want to withdraw and retreat into themselves when experiencing negative emotions from others rather than trying to interact or help out of a desire to please. If there is no response from adults in their life, they may even act out on their own feelings in order to get attention.

2. Sensitive to noises

These children are startled easily as babies and are still easily startled as adults. They may be distracted by noise, seem to hear things that aren't there, and often seem hyper-aware.

3. Sensitive to light

Due to increased sensory processing, a highly sensitive child is more aware of the subtleties of light, shadow, color. This can lead to excessive tear production in response to bright lights or fluorescent lights.

4. Sensitive to clothing

Children who have a highly sensitive temperament tend to be highly aware of their physical surroundings. This awareness extends to their clothing, and they are typically sensitive to the texture or weight of different types of fabrics, as well as the clothes themselves being too tight, loose, heavy, or light.

5. Sensitive to scents

In addition to being easily overwhelmed by the smells of perfumes, colognes, gasoline, cleaning products, air fresheners, and smoke, many highly sensitive children find smells that are barely noticeable to most people bothersome. For these children wearing certain types of clothes can be a real problem.

6. Dislike change

Prefer close relationships.

7. Hard on themselves

Children who are highly sensitive have a low tolerance for mistakes and are hard on themselves when they do something wrong.

8. Overly-worried about what others think

CHAPTER 4:

Symptoms of Anxiety in Children

Anxiety can have a number of symptoms in children. From feeling too much stress to trouble with sleeping, anxiety can affect kids in many ways. These are some of the most common symptoms.

- Finding it hard to concentrate.
- Not sleeping, or waking in the night with bad dreams.
- Not eating properly.
- Quickly getting angry or irritable and being out of control during outbursts.
- Constantly worrying or having negative thoughts.
- Feeling tense and fidgety or using the toilet often.

These are some of the most common symptoms of anxiety in children. Sometimes these symptoms can mean other things, too. If your child has any of these symptoms, talk to your doctor about whether they could be caused by anxiety. Your child will get a physical exam as well as a mental health check to help find out what is causing the symptoms.

Sensitivity and Intelligence

Sensitivity toward beauty, people, places, and one's environment is a common characteristic of intelligent people. Some studies have shown that gifted adults express a high level of sensitivity due to their superior aesthetic abilities. Aesthetic sensitivity is a trait that gifted children share with adults. It is a relative concept, meaning that the aesthetic sensitivity of people can be high, low, or medium. According to the findings provided by the studies done by Brown and Plaud in 2004 and Hewitt et al. in 2008, gifted children tend to have higher levels of sensitivity compared to their non-gifted peers. These results also suggest that highly sensitive persons are more likely to possess creative abilities and superior cognitive skills. The concept of aesthetic sensitivity was developed from studies on personality psychology as well as on identifying the strengths gifted individuals possess compared to their counterparts with a lower level of giftedness (Hembree & Lawing, 2007; Lopez et al., 2009).

Aesthetic sensitivity can be seen as part of the giftedness concept. According to Vetter (1983), giftedness is the result of an interaction between a number of factors: hereditary, environmental, and structural alterations in cognitive processing abilities. These possible changes in cognitive processing abilities are also likely to affect a person's ability to perceive and understand his environment. Gifted individuals are more sensitive than others to the environment and are able to process information better than others due to their heightened perceptiveness (Hembree & Lawing, 2007; Lopez et al., 2009).

According to Flynn (2001), there is an inverse relationship between intelligence and aesthetic sensitivity. Less intelligent people have lower levels of aesthetic sensitivity. This may be because they are not able to perceive or understand the environment as well as their more intelligent counterparts. Flynn also posits that there are both positive and negative relationships between intelligence and sensitivity, depending on the domain (Flynn & Torrey, 2002). He explains that in domains where individuals often make mistakes (such as in sports), intelligence can reduce a person's sensitivity to mistakes they make. On the other hand, in domains that require careful perception (such as art and science), intelligence may increase a person's level of aesthetic sensitivity.

Studies done by Hewitt et al. (2008) used the Scholastic Aptitude Test (SAT) and the Wonderlic Personnel Test (WPT) data to classify the dependent variable's distribution into different groups. The studies showed that individuals who had high levels of intelligence also had higher levels of aesthetic sensitivity compared to those with lower levels of intelligence. In addition, many skills and abilities play important roles in aesthetic sensitivity, such as cognitive abilities such as working memory, attention, and reading fluency. From this point of view, aesthetic sensitivity can be viewed as an indicator of one's intelligence (Hembree & Lawing, 2007). Aesthetic sensitivity is an aspect of intelligence because it can be seen as a cognitive ability that has the power to shape one's perception of the environment (Brown & Plaud, 2004; Flynn, 2001). Research studies that include neurophysiological and neuropsychological tests have shown that aesthetic sensitivity and intelligence are related through certain brain mechanisms. Two different views of aesthetic sensitivity: the Big Five Model and the Sensitivity Theory, have been used to study how individuals process information. The Big Five Model shows five dimensions for describing all possible traits: Openness to Experience and Conscientiousness (low-high), Agreeableness, Extraversion, and Emotional Stability (negative-positive). The Sensitivity Theory also contains five dimensions, and its research has been conducted in different domains such as health, art, and psychology.

The Big Five Model posits that individuals with high levels of aesthetic sensitivity are more likely to be creative and to apply unusual perspectives. Both of these traits have positive effects on the person, especially in the domains of science and technology (Brown & Plaud, 2004; Flynn, 2001). In addition to scientific research studies that involved neuropsychological tests, case studies have shown similar results about aesthetic sensitivity and the Big Five model. Specifically, case study analysis showed that gifted children tended to have high levels of aesthetic sensitivity compared to their non-gifted counterparts (Brown & Plaud, 2004). Some studies also showed that highly sensitive children are likely to have creative abilities and superior cognitive skills (Hembree & Lawing, 2007).

As for the Sensitivity Theory, which is based on the Sensation-Intuition-Sensation (SIS) theory, it holds that aesthetic sensitivity may be characterized by six dimensions. The six dimensions are the intensity of perception, response to the perceptual experience, sensitivity to the physical beauty of objects and their detail with respect to abstract qualities, appreciation for art and music in terms of its unique qualities, and emotional/mental aspects (Brown & Plaud, 2004).

The factors that influence aesthetic sensitivity include biological factors such as personality and intelligence. An individual's personality affects their perception of beauty. The more developed an individual's personality is, the more likely he or she is to explore and be interested in other areas of life (Brown & Plaud, 2004; Flynn, 2001). Aesthetic sensitivity can also be influenced by intelligence. Flynn's (2001) theory states that aesthetic sensitivity is a subcomponent of intelligence, and it has been proven through neuropsychological tests. This means that individuals with higher levels of intelligence are more likely to have higher levels of cognitive ability, thus increasing their level of aesthetic sensitivity.

Aesthetic sensitivity contributes to one's development in many ways. It enhances one's aesthetic experience and the way one perceives the environment. It is also important for one's ability to pick up on subtleties in a visual sense. Since aesthetic sensitivity is an inter-related concept, it is vital to understand the differences between sensitivity and preference. The main difference between the two comes from their relationship with others. A person who perceives objects differently than others can feel a deep connection or attachment to those objects (Reed & Irwin, 2000). The term "preference" refers to the individual interest in the object (Reed & Irwin, 2000). However, when someone perceives an object as pleasurable, they are picking up on another person's preferences. When this person translates that information in a way that is not related to their personal desires, they begin to develop an aesthetic sensitivity.

Aesthetics can be expanded to other fields such as music, art, and architecture. However, "aesthetic" is commonly used to describe the beauty or appreciation of those things relating to concepts such as color and beauty in nature. This definition of aesthetic has been adopted into many different cultures and languages (Reed & Irwin, 2000). The development of aesthetics starts at an early age. Babies respond differently depending on their level of exposure to objects such as bright lights or soft textures (Reed & Irwin, 2000). For example, babies with darker skin tones grow up to perceive trade-in colors. They also show a preference for soft textures and do not respond as much to color. In the 1960s, an art critic and theorist named Clement Greenberg discovered that there was beauty in what he called "the language of the gestalt"—namely, empty space or mere outline (Crowther & Lampe, 2005). Greenberg's theory led him to question whether it was possible for aesthetic judgment to be objective. He rejected the possibility of aesthetic judgments being based solely on personal experience or preference because he believed that such judgments were subjectively formed and, therefore, flawed

(Crowther & Lampe, 2005). He also rejected the notion of aesthetic values being based purely on emotions. Instead, he proposed that art can be seen as an expression of a culture's moral values.

Greenberg believed that artistic excellence is the result of a synthesis of two processes:

1. An artist's ability to express
2. Culture's ability to comprehend what is expressed

To put it another way, these two processes are necessary but not sufficient conditions for aesthetic excellence (Crowther & Lampe, 2005). Greenberg's theory, while interesting, has been criticized in recent years. Critics of Greenberg's theory propose that art is subjective and does not require both the artist and the audience to be familiar with an "objective" culture (Takahashi et al., 2007).

Greenberg's theory has also been criticized for failing to take into account the importance of other aesthetic qualities such as color and music (Takahashi et al., 2007). There is currently no consensus on what makes an art object "beautiful." However, most researchers of aesthetics agree that there are many factors that can influence an individual's perception of beauty. Such factors are related to a person's culture and personal experience. Aesthetic preferences may have a significant impact on an individual's mental health.

A study done by Tattersall and Byng (1984) sought to determine whether aesthetic preferences had any implications for mental health. The study included 135 participants between the ages of 18 to 25. The participants were all asked to list their favorite music, TV programs, movies, songs, and plays from various countries across the world, including the UK, USA, Canada, Italy, and Germany. The researchers then compared the preferences of their participants and found that more than half of the participants in each sample had a single favorite category. Most of these individuals had a preference for one specific kind of music, TV program, or movie. Furthermore, the researchers found that aesthetic preferences were positively related to self-rated mental health and well-being but negatively related to self-rated physical health (Tattersall & Byng, 1984).

Aesthetic sensitivity has been found to have an impact on one's intelligence. Studies have also shown that people with high levels of intelligence are more likely to be creative than those with lower levels (Brown & Plaud, 2004; Flynn, 2001). Flynn (2001) has proposed his theory regarding the relationship between intelligence and aesthetic sensitivity. He believes that aesthetic sensitivity is a subcomponent of intelligence. Intelligence is a very broad concept that refers to one's ability to pick up on cues in one's environment (Brown & Plaud, 2004). Flynn argues that because individuals with higher levels of intelligence are able to perceive and understand the environment better, they are more likely to have higher levels of aesthetic sensitivity as well.

Aesthetic sensitivity can be seen as a form of intelligence because it allows an individual to pick up on subtle cues in their environment (Brown & Plaud, 2004). Women, on average, are more likely to be more sensitive to their environment than men (Flynn, 2001). Flynn describes this as a quicker form of intelligence. This may partially be because women are always aware that they are being observed and tend to display their emotions more often (Flynn, 2001).

Creative individuals can have a greater impact on our lives than non-creative people who may not have the ability to extrapolate from their surroundings. There are many examples of individuals who apply unusual perspectives to their surroundings, for example, artists and scientists.

In terms of the relationship between aesthetic sensitivity and intelligence, this branch of psychology is just starting to be studied. It has been shown that there is a positive correlation between both variables (Brown & Plaud, 2004). The Big Five model has the advantage of being able to control for a large number of variables. This provides solid evidence that aesthetic sensitivity is a subcomponent of intelligence (Hembree & Lawing, 2007). The Sensitivity Theory supports this finding in that it shows that the relationship between both variables is not limited to one particular domain or experience (Brown & Plaud, 2004).

Sensitivity may be composed of many different components, including cognitive abilities such as working memory and attention. Studies have shown that individuals who have a higher level of intelligence also tend to perform better on tests, such as the digit span test and the Raven's Coloured Progressive Matrices Test (Reed et al., 2007).

Cognitive scientists in the field of cognitive aesthetics study the nature of perceptual and emotional experiences, the cognitive bases of these experiences, and their role in aesthetic preferences. More specifically, researchers in this field conduct empirical research to understand if activation in certain brain regions is correlated with preferences for various kinds of artistic styles, such as Impressionist art. The discipline was founded by George Lakoff and Mark Johnson's "Metaphors We Lived By" (1980) and was introduced to a larger theoretical audience by Denis Dutton's article "The Art Instinct" for "The New York Times Magazine" (2001).

The paradigm of cognitive aesthetics has also been applied to technological design and medical treatment, such as at the Stanford School of Design. Cognitive aesthetics also lies on the basis of several computational models for generating visual art. The resulting applications range from the adaptive collage art generator PictoCue to fractal art renderers like Apollonian Fractal. In addition, cognitive approaches to aesthetics have informed research in computational creativity, which attempts to develop computer programs that can autonomously create highly creative works of art, music, or other cultural artifacts. Exploring the psychology of art, and especially painting, has been an interest of psychologists since the time of Leonardo da Vinci.

Modern academic programs in psychology are sometimes the result of collaboration between artists and psychiatrists or psychoanalysts. For example, Sigmund Freud's "Introductory Lectures on Psychoanalysis" (1916–17) was originally developed to teach physicians how to use psychoanalysis to treat patients suffering from mental disorders, many of whom were artists or musicians. Likewise, some modern art schools have invited clinical psychologists or psychoanalysts to teach workshops on personality development in artists and students as well as art therapy. As well, many popular psychology books are written by authors who are artists or whose work involves visual representations. For example, Carl Jung wrote "The Psychology of Art" (1919) to explore subjects such as the psychology of art in relation to symbolism and the unconscious, while more recently, Barbara Fredrickson has written "Positivity: Overcoming the Negative Self and Changing Your Mind for Good" to explore positive psychology in relation to creativity and well-being.

In film studies, aesthetics encompasses all visual elements of filmmaking. Though very few films are aesthetically perfect, artistic expression can be said to exist at all levels of filmmaking. The level of craftsmanship in the visual aspects of filmmaking affects the audience's response to a film. In television studies, aesthetic choices are those made in the design and production of a television show. An "aesthetic" is defined as an emotional effect that is evoked by both visual and aural elements. Aesthetic choices may refer to:

In video game studies, aesthetic choices are those made in the design and production of a video game. The academic study of video game aesthetics is closely related to game studies, which includes ludology, narratology, new media, and many other approaches. Aesthetics is a branch of philosophy and often intersects with other academic disciplines such as art history, architecture, linguistics, religion, and history. Aesthetics is generally applied to the appreciation of visual art. However, it can also refer to the appreciation of oral or written texts or musical works. In this sense, aesthetics is closely related to criticism, which can be seen as a subset of aesthetics.

In the West since classical antiquity (see ancient Greek philosophy), philosophy has been strongly influenced by aesthetic theories in Plato and Aristotle (see "The Theory of Forms"), especially their discussions about beauty and its role in thinking. In the 19th century, Kant and Hegel developed the study of aesthetics as a discipline. In modern times, Western philosophy of art has been called "aesthetics," and it is commonly divided into three categories: classical aesthetics, phenomenological aesthetics, and hermeneutic aesthetics. Classical aesthetics (see Aristotle) is concerned with the nature of art, beauty, and the artist's role in society. It examines the question, "What is a work of art?" Aristotle offers two answers: a material and an ideal one. The ideal answer involves perceiving the work as it is in itself, as a unity of form and matter. The material answer places emphasis on that which makes up the work of art: shape, occupation of space, movement, or language.

The creation of beautiful objects is one goal, but so too is their appreciation by other human beings. Phenomenological aesthetics, led by theorists like Maurice Merleau-Ponty, deals with the way objects are perceived in a manner that makes them more than just material. One aim is to understand the role that our physical being plays in shaping our experience of objects. In contrast to classical aesthetics, phenomenological aesthetics tends to focus on the uniqueness of each perception and its ability to elicit responses from an emotional and intellectual unconscious. It's a subjective aesthetic that focuses on how art can make us feel and relate to different aspects of human experience instead of creating logic or rationality

Essentially, phenomenology sees perception as an active process. It's in this sense that understanding art has to do with one's ability to be sensitive and receptive to the aesthetic experience. Hermeneutic aesthetics (see Heidegger; Gadamer), also called "interpretive aesthetics" or "philosophical hermeneutics," is the study of interpretation in response to products of human making such as art, literature, film, architecture, and music. Hermeneutics questions what a text means beyond its literal surface meaning due to its embedded cultural context. The study of hermeneutics is closely tied with philosophical questions about the experience of art itself. Philosophers Karl Löwith (1899–1982) and Hans Georg Gadamer (1900–2002) are the most prominent figures in the 20th century who have dealt with aesthetic experience.

Gadamer's book, "The Aesthetic Problem," extends the scope of aesthetics beyond art to include other human creations. Since his work, philosophers, such as Robert C. Solomon in "Aesthetics" and "The Concealed Art of Painting: An Essay on Kantian Aesthetics," have taken up the study of aesthetics as a consistent philosophical subject in its own right. Gadamer did not use the term "aesthetics" to describe his philosophical approach, preferring instead to speak of a "hermeneutics of art." His reflections, however, have inspired many methodologies for interpreting and analyzing works of art; indeed, his work helped to revive the interest in aesthetics as a whole. Gadamer's influence is also evident in contemporary hermeneutical aesthetics and theories such as those of Michael Murray.

There are various ways that one can approach the definition of aesthetics. One way is by identifying the definition of art and its relationship with aesthetics. In the arts, aesthetics is often viewed as the study of a work's form, content, and effects on an audience. This view has been popular for such works as paintings, music, and sculptures. It is believed that a work's content is shaped by historical context and individual perspective. For instance, Beethoven's 9th Symphony could have different meanings to an audience in China than it would for a U.S. audience. Individual differences in perception can also influence one's understanding of a certain work; for example, how one person interprets Picasso's painting "Guernica" can differ from another person's interpretation of the same painting. Therefore, aesthetics is the study of the way individuals who view a certain work perceive it and its meaning. A paradigmatic example of this is Marcel Duchamp's readymades or "La Mariée mise à nu par ses célibataires, même" (The Bride Stripped Bare by Her Bachelors, Even), which is among the most influential works in 20th-century art as well as one of the earliest examples of conceptual art. Duchamp claims that it was not until his creation of "Fountain," a mass-produced urinal signed "R. Mutt," that he began thinking about what constitutes an object to be considered art. The one-time urinal now resides in the permanent collection of New York's Museum of Modern Art. Duchamp's Fountain is a simple porcelain urinal, available from a hardware store that was adapted by the artist into a work of art. In doing so, Duchamp redefined the very nature of art and questioned its definition. Rather than deriving an item's artistic relevance from its inherent cultural value or monetary significance, he derived it from its aesthetic standing as it pertains to everyday life.

Aesthetics can be defined as the study and criticism of these objects based on their form, content, and effects on an audience. In his book "Art, Intention, and Reason in the Philosophy of Arthur Danto," Arthur C. Danto discusses how aesthetics relates to art-making and criticism. He claims that there is a major difference between the way historians of art perceive and make sense of an artwork and the way that the artist or critic perceives and makes sense of a work. As he puts it, "In the production or criticism of art, we are not dealing with an internalized set of signs but with an item on a par with other things in the world." For example, when looking at Michelangelo's statue David, one must take into account its form, subject matter, medium (i.e., marble), and historical context in order to make sense of it; however, when the artist or critic views the sculpture, they do not need to take into account these same elements. Thus, Danto suggests that when looking at a work of art, we must go beyond the items of which an artwork consists in order to take into account its aesthetic nature. Understood in this way, aesthetics is defined as the analysis and critique of aesthetic objects.

Aesthetics deals with individual tastes and opinions. Some critics state that there are underlying facts and laws governing artistic works but no simple general principles of aesthetics. The necessity for aesthetic judgment is often stressed: without it, there can be no art criticism. It is also argued that there are ethical and moral aspects to aesthetic evaluation. Aesthetics is our concern for the sensory appearances of things. The branch of philosophy called aesthetics studies the nature of beauty, art, and taste, with the creation and appreciation of beauty. Aesthetics has traditionally been described as a sub-category of philosophy that deals with the nature of art and beauty. This definition is somewhat broad because it encompasses both science (formal science in particular) and humanities such as music, painting, sculpture, photography, literature/poetry, and drama. However, the discipline and its subject matter can be more narrowly described as studies of the nature of art and beauty in relation to their communication effects. Aesthetics is also closely related to art criticism. Aesthetics concerns itself with such areas of study as:

Aesthetic perception studies the way people see things so as to be able to appreciate them more fully or differently, and often it is said that the experience of beauty expresses our particular understanding of what beauty is. This idea has inspired many authors who have written about aesthetics in English, from Plato (427–347) onwards; they have helped create a guiding framework for thinking about art which has been called Kantian aesthetics. Kant's work on aesthetics is designed to investigate humans' response to beauty, and more immediately, to attempt to establish a set of concrete criteria that will allow them to define what is "beautiful" and see how that leads to other concepts in aesthetics. Kantian aesthetics also considers the so-called disinterested attitude, which asks whether art is worthwhile if it does not convey a purpose or message. Kant thinks that there are three questions within aesthetic theory:

Because Kantian aesthetics focuses on beauty, it can be considered a branch of philosophy. However, this definition is broad because it encompasses thoughts and feelings about art in general rather than specifically about fine arts such as painting or sculpture. Moreover, Kant did not specifically discuss what is now called aesthetics but the concept of aesthetic experience. In this sense, aesthetics can be studied either as a subset of pure philosophy or as a subset of practical philosophy; however, Kant was much more interested in discussing art and literature in relation to human nature. While Kantian aesthetics is still highly influential today, current aesthetic theories go beyond Kantian ideas. This evolution began in Germany and Austria when theorists began putting forth the idea that viewers may respond to an artwork based on their own personal feelings and preferences; this is known as subjectivism (the theory that beauty depends on the response of the beholder). The chief proponent of this theory was Friedrich Schiller. In addition to an emphasis on the subjective nature of aesthetic evaluation, Schiller also argued that there was a distinction between art and beauty (aesthetic value). According to this theory, beauty is based on form and harmony in works of art, while art is based on the expression of its message. Another German aesthetician who tried to push aesthetics out of the realm of "pure philosophy" was Heinrich Wölfflin (1864–1945); he developed his own version of Kantian aesthetics due to his interest in formal analysis rather than practical content. He claimed that beauty could be expressed in different ways, so he focused on analyzing its various forms: musical composition and painting. Wölfflin claimed that, while two works of art may both have beautiful forms, they could not be judged to be equally beautiful. His methods became a widespread model in the field of art history, and his ideas influenced some other philosophers as well. The concept of subjectivism also inspired the "aesthetics of presence" philosophy (also known as existentialist aesthetics), which argued that beauty should be seen as an experience rather than a rational understanding; this idea was put forth by Peter Kivy in "The Corded Shell" (1969)

While Kantian aesthetics focused on beauty and the experience of beauty, aesthetic theories have expanded to include other aspects of artistic and literary works. Kant believed that people should be able to find beauty in all works of art, but aesthetics have been more widely debated since the mid-20th century. This debate involved both sides arguing that there are certain circumstances under which aesthetic value cannot be found in the work of art: these are called formalist objections to art. Some critics claim that the way people enjoy works of art is subjective; therefore, there are no objective standards for judging them. They claim that because beauty is in the eye of the beholder, what makes a painting beautiful is entirely dependent on the person looking at it. Another issue in modern aesthetic theory is whether or not there are any objective standards for evaluating works of art (as proposed by Aristotle in his Poetics).

The disagreement over issues like these has prompted literary theorists to argue that there are universal laws of aesthetics; they argue that there are objective standards by which people can judge how the arts should be evaluated (as Thomas MacFarland has done with "The Aesthetic"). Moreover, critics have discussed the role of language when discussing art and literature. In his book "Culture, Media, Language," Roland Barthes argued that language has an effect on the way in which we perceive objects. Aesthetics deals with different ways in which people can experience beauty. It is important to note that people do not all experience beauty in the same way and that one's aesthetic experience depends heavily on one's own background. For instance, one person may think a Van Gogh painting is beautiful because it makes them feel calm and peaceful, while another person may simply be bored by it. This is because there are many different meanings of beauty, and beauty varies from culture to culture.

There are also many different ways that one can experience beauty. A person may feel that a painting is beautiful because it makes them feel peaceful or calm but may think it is bad art because the artist did not accurately depict the piece. Another cause for the difference in one's aesthetic experience is the setting in which art is viewed. In a museum, people look at beautiful paintings in silence, whereas on an airplane, people are able to view them while being rushed by turbulence. This causes people to be able to appreciate the paintings differently because of how they view them, no matter where they are. Aesthetic experiences can also differ based on how one was raised. Some people may view a house of horrors as beautiful because they were raised as a horror film fan, whereas others may find the attraction grotesque. People can also view art differently if they have experienced similar things before. If someone has never seen or heard of Picasso before, they will not recognize his work as that of an artist, but if they had already studied about him in school, they would then know his work for what it is. This is because people associate certain ideas with certain experiences, and their perception is based on this association; thus, the meaning differs from person to person based on how the person connects experiences and ideas to each other.

The development of aesthetics can be divided into periods. In the ancient Greek world, there was a lot of aesthetic activity. However, ideas of beauty changed drastically with the times. For instance, in Egyptian times, it was believed that humans were made out of mud and dirt; thus, the ideal human body was composed entirely of mud and dust. In the 1950s through 1960s in America, people began to think differently about beauty; they began thinking that beauty came from all different types of life forms—from animals to insects as well as humans. Aesthetics is also related to the history of art criticism (art criticism).

Around 2,500 years ago in Ancient Greece (1600–1200 BC), there were three different ways to speak about aesthetics that are still used today. Beauty was defined as "the splendor of truth," "the splendor of form," and "the mode of good." These three terms are still important in aesthetic theory today. Over time different views about beauty emerged.

In Ancient Greece, from around the 6th century BC, beauty started to be seen less as a formal quality and more as the manifestation of divine spiritual power; thus, it was believed that the gods had made each thing beautiful. This view was supported by Western philosophers such as Immanuel Kant (1724–1804), who claimed that the human mind plays a central role in esthetic experience.

The 19th century brought the idea that people are affected by beauty, even if they do not realize it. Different types of art were analyzed to see how they make an impression on the observer. Charles Baudelaire (1821–1867), in his "The Painter of Modern Life," argued that human behavior is strongly influenced by the imperceptible or subliminal effects of beauty; thus, the decorative arts influence society more than one might think.

In the 20th century, theories about aesthetics became more complicated, and they tried to integrate a variety of cultural factors into their analyses. For example, Philip Johnson (1906–2001) argued that the style of the work of art depends on the culture in which it is seen and that there are differences between "beautifully designed" objects and those that are "merely nicely done." For instance, religious objects are not judged to be as aesthetically pleasing as pleasant-to-the-eye objects such as furniture or jewelry. Furthermore, you cannot judge a painting because it looks beautiful, but according to what something has to say; thus, a painting can be considered aesthetically appealing even if it does not look beautiful. Arthur Danto (b. 1928) distinguished between the "aesthetic attitude" and the "aesthetic experience." According to Danto, something can be considered art if it generates an aesthetic attitude. Thus, a piece of art is not judged according to its beauty alone; instead, it is judged according to how its meaning has been conveyed through its aesthetic attitude.

Aesthetics is related to art criticism because critics do not merely describe what they see in an artwork, but instead, they judge it. The aesthetic theory tries to define principles, criteria, or standards by which works of art are judged. An example would be Kant's "Critique of Judgment," in which he analyzes beauty and the respective judgment involved in perception. He distinguishes between judgments of "taste," which are subjective, and judgments of "discursive" or "rational" understanding, which are supposedly objective. In addition, aesthetic theories in the 20th century also explored the notion of "meaningful beauty" (or "aesthetic meaning")—the extent to which an artwork conveys a message. For example, Carl Jung (1875–1961) argues that artists should not be afraid to ask themselves: "Does this drawing express a certain idea?" Artists who adhere to this ideal are thus seen as communicating their own personal messages to the viewer. Similarly, according to Kant's teachings, there is the need for humans to look beyond just beauty when assessing art; it must also be judged against other standards such as morality and rationality, which Kant believed was impossible for works of art and art criticism.

Aesthetics has also been applied to the study of literature. The branch of aesthetics dealing with literature is called narratology, and it focuses on how literary texts create specific effects. In this view, narratives are analyzed in terms of the values they promote and the emotions they elicit from their readers. In addition to theories about narrative meaning, there are also those that focus on how literary works affect their readers emotionally. For example, Roland Barthes (1915–1980) argues that a novel is not only a story but also an image that "produces a reality." Narrative aesthetics is concerned with how literary narratives achieve their effects. In this approach, the aesthetic values of a narrative are not limited to its literary qualities, and instead, the impact a narrative has on its readers is examined. Thus, writers create narratives with the intention of affecting their readers' emotions in order to achieve particular effects. Nelson Goodman (1906–1998), for example, argues that texts have the ability to compel their audience into a particular way of thinking by providing them with what he calls "rhetorical situations" (or "rhetorical forms").

The use of language for various rhetorical purposes is an important feature of many narratives; thus, it can be assumed that there are certain types of discourse that are more effective than others. In this approach, scholars focus on how it can be used to impart ideological values. For instance, in his work "The Languages of Art," Claude Lévi-Strauss (1908–2009) argues that the use of poetic language can be used to create a particular effect.

Many aesthetic theories have also been applied to the study of literature in terms of their literary representation; it is important to note that literary representation is not solely based on descriptions but rather involves the characters' actions as well as their thoughts and feelings. In this approach, scholars examine characters' actions and motives in order to determine how they are depicted through literary texts. For example, in his book "The Poetics of Plot," literary critic Wayne C. Booth (1921–2005) argues that stories do not merely depict characters and their actions but also the reasons why they act the way they do. Thus, a story's plot is formed from its characters' thoughts and feelings as well as their actions. This is significant in the field of narrative aesthetics because it creates moral dilemmas for readers to think about, thus prompting them to reflect upon what they personally would do in a similar situation. Aesthetics has been used to analyze different types of art such as painting, sculpture, and architecture.

These fields share similar definitions and principles regarding what constitutes beauty, but they do have different methods of analysis. For example, for architecture, aesthetics focuses on the formal beauty of the building, such as its shape or its decoration. Certain types of art are also analyzed in terms of their forms. For example, in his book "Form and Meaning," architectural theorist Paolo Soleri (1922–2007) argues that buildings need to be able to communicate a feeling of presence and reality; thus, he gives special significance to a building's ability to focus on meaning rather than form. Aesthetic theories have also been used to analyze music. For example, a composer's work can be judged by how it makes an audience feel. Thus, artistic merit may depend on whether or not the work is capable of arousing an appropriate emotion (such as sadness) in the audience. Aesthetics also overlaps with musical analysis, which is concerned with how music sounds (for example, in terms of its tone color).

There are two different types of musical analysis—analyzing music through language and analyzing it through numbers. The former is associated with writers such as Heinrich Schenker (1868–1935), and the latter is associated with theorists such as Allen Forte (with his pitch-class set theory). Aesthetics is also associated with the study of aesthetics in other areas such as technology and art history. For example, in the field of art history, it is a common method for researchers to apply aesthetic theories to works of art that they analyze. In this approach, the "aesthetic experience" that one has looked at in an artwork is now examined. Aesthetics can also be used when analyzing current trends in certain fields and their future directions (for example, in terms of technological progress). According to scholar Erick Jenkins (b. 1949), this approach is based on the idea that "the continued use of older technologies results in aesthetic decline" (such as the "decline of graphic design in favor of computer graphics"). The concept of design relates to aesthetics. For example, in his book "Design as Art," Chen-Bo Zhong (b. 1961) discusses the idea that a form needs to be beautiful or not, but also that it should have a certain degree of function and efficiency. He argues that form and function are inseparable; thus, two objects cannot simply be considered beautiful if their form is unacceptable (for example, a square circle). In the study of design, many scholars use aesthetic theory to analyze and judge objects. For instance, in his critique titled "Aesthetics and Design," designer Nigel Cross (b. 1936) argues that aesthetics is not an intrinsic quality of a product; instead, it is something that is created through knowledge of craftsmanship and understanding of the material that has been used.

Aesthetics can be studied from a philosophical point of view through different disciplines, including art history, philosophy, and psychology. Since aesthetics relies on its relationship with other fields such as art criticism and rhetoric (the systematic study of writing), one can also study its historical development in order to determine how it has changed over time. For example, it can be analyzed according to what philosophers have said about it throughout history, as well as their different aesthetic theories. The history of aesthetics spans over two thousand years. During this period, there have been many debates on what makes something beautiful; an important question has always been whether a thing is beautiful because of its form or because of its function (this was debated by Kant). Aesthetics has also been applied to a wide range of topics, such as the perception of art and literature and the psychological effect that these can cause. In contemporary times, the term is used in a variety of contexts; for example, aesthetics are now applied to everyday objects such as cars and appliances. In addition, it is often used in fields such as product design, in which an object is created with its "aesthetic qualities" in mind. According to the philosopher Miles Burnyeat, it is difficult to provide a succinct definition of aesthetics because there are so many different theories about what it is. In his essay "Aesthetics and Anaesthetics," he wrote: "One might almost as well try to single out something called 'physics'—as if there were one thing called 'physics' that was used by physicists."

Similarly, in his essay titled "Aesthetics," Richard Wollheim (b. 1910) stated that there are "two diametrically opposed ways of thinking about aesthetics." According to Wollheim, some thinkers view aesthetics as a science of forms, and others view it as the study of material objects; he compared these two approaches as "the two poles" of aesthetics.

Critic Harold Bloom (1933–2013) defined aesthetics as a "disciplined understanding and appreciation of beauty."

Aristotle, in his book "Rhetoric," argued that the purpose of creating rhetoric was to educate the audience; thus, rhetoric should be used to illustrate the best possible course of action. In this view, aesthetics is considered an important aspect because it validates this course of action. Furthermore, according to Aristotle, rhetoric works through persuading an audience to choose one action over another; thus, it is also seen as an important feature of aesthetics.

The Italian philosopher Giorgio Agamben (b. 1942) draws parallels between aesthetics and ethics, seeing both as a way of evaluating human life. Thus, he argues that aesthetics and ethics are inseparable concepts because they are both concerned with how people live their lives. In his work "The Open," he explains this by stating, "Aesthetics is the ontology of existence, ethics its teleology." He also argues that aesthetics has an ethical dimension; for example, when beauty is defined, it also contains a particular moral position.

According to philosopher Paul Ricoeur (1913–2005), the concept of beauty is a moral issue. Drawing on his works "The Symbolism of Evil" and "L'Avant-Garde," he argues that there are certain things that are considered beautiful and which are not; this vision of beauty could be seen as a description of what is morally right or wrong. In his work "The Conflict of Interpretations: Themes from the Phenomenology of Life," Ricoeur states that "aesthetic appreciation presupposes moral judgment." There are two different approaches to aesthetics—aesthetic criticism and aesthetic theory. Aesthetic criticism is the practice of judging a work of art and making a verbal or written assessment about its aesthetic value. The aim of aesthetic criticism is to explain what makes a particular thing beautiful in terms of its form and function. In order to achieve this, many writers have emphasized the importance of examining works from different perspectives; thus, it can be assumed that there are certain features of an object that need to be examined in detail. For example, in his essay "On Beauty," the English philosopher Roger Scruton (b. 1944) states that beauty can be found through examining two things—the "formal" and "material"; he uses these terms mainly in reference to sensory properties such as color, shape, and texture.

Another approach to aesthetics is the aesthetic theory, which focuses on what is aesthetically valuable about a work of art. Scholars have used the term "ethical" to describe the various ways in which works of art and literature communicate moral values. An example would be literature that deals with corruption, such as Robert Louis Stevenson's novel "The Strange Case of Dr. Jekyll and Mr. Hyde." This novel contains elements that the author described as an "objectionable" but "moral" story. Another example is in Hans Christian Andersen's (1805–1875) fairy tale "The Emperor's New Clothes"; here, the moral issue is about vanity and its consequences.

Literary critic Wayne C. Booth (1921–2005) argues that stories do not simply depict characters and actions, but also the reasons why they act the way they do; thus, a story's plot is formed from its characters' thoughts and feelings as well as their actions. This has been termed a "narrative aesthetics." For example, Shakespeare's play "Hamlet" has been described as a play where the moral and aesthetic issues are inseparable. There are many trends in ethical aesthetics that reflect the concerns of society; for instance, there has been an increase in contemporary issues which are increasingly being reflected in art and literature. For instance, the artist Damien Hirst (b. 1965) often uses his work to comment on political events such as war and capitalism; thus, his works can be seen as containing an element of ethical morality. Similarly, the magician David Blaine's (b. 1973) art is meant to challenge how people view life and death; he describes his controversial performance artworks as "modern-day morality tales." Another example is the work of the novelist and playwright Martin Amis (b. 1949); his novels contain themes such as class conflict and terrorism.

The aesthetic theories of Immanuel Kant (1724–1804) have been influential on aesthetics to the present day. The German philosopher believed that beauty is a property of an object, but only when what it signifies is not in conflict with its form. In other words, if an object's aesthetic properties are not in conflict with its meaning, then it is considered beautiful. Kant's theory of beauty was based mainly on his theory of art and is described as a "formalist" model. He assumed that there are two parts that make up an artwork—the form of an object and its function; the purpose for which an object was designed is also part of what determines its aesthetic value. Kant believed that beauty was inextricably linked to morality, logic, and science; according to Kant, art has three main functions—art is a means of expressing our human psychology and subjectivity, a medium for philosophical thought, and an aesthetic object with artistic properties. It is stressed that Kant's view of aesthetics was based on his teleological view of art, which means that the artist produces beauty through the use of their specialized skills and artistic ability rather than by chance.

The German philosopher Arthur Schopenhauer (1788–1860) was interested in aesthetics as it related to religion, morality, and the human body. According to literary critic David Simpson (b. 1939), Schopenhauer saw aesthetic experiences as a means of "spiritual uplift." For example, in his book "On Aesthetic Education," he describes how many people can be brought closer to God when they feel beauty; he also gives examples from everyday life using food as a common example. Simpson goes on to argue that this view of aesthetics as spiritual guidance can be applied to a number of issues, such as gender relations and sexuality. Schopenhauer was also interested in the concept of "the ugly." He believed that the experience of ugliness was an important and necessary part of aesthetic appreciation; thus, he used ugliness as a philosophical term for what is ugly and unpleasant. He stated that the experience of the ugly is an "ethical" means of understanding aesthetic concepts.

The German philosopher Wilhelm Windelband (1848–1915) was influenced by Kant's ideas and developed his own approach to aesthetics; he believed that aesthetics is concerned with the "critique of taste" and was less interested in the object itself than in how it is judged. For example, he argued that art criticism should examine whether a painting is successful or not; thus, there are two aspects to aesthetics—the "subjective" and the "objective." Windelband believed that Kant's approach was too simplistic; for example, when discussing the concept of beauty, Kant described it as having a property of being felt "independently" from its circumstances. This view was rejected by Windelband because he believed that beauty is "intrinsically" connected to the perceiver; otherwise, it would only be a concept in the mind of the viewer. This approach was based on Kant's belief that if all art were understood in terms of meaning, then it would be impossible to distinguish between art and what cannot be called art.

Aesthetic psychology refers to attempts to understand how people experience aesthetic pleasures such as pleasure in art or music. The aesthetics of aesthetics has been criticized as being an unwarranted discipline that lacks an adequate methodology; according to philosopher Peter Strawson (1917–2009), it is defined by its inability to provide any evidence for its claims. The questions of aesthetics were traditionally considered to be a branch of philosophy, but with the development of various new disciplines (such as cultural studies, psychology, and sociology), the study of aesthetics has expanded into those new areas.

CHAPTER 5:

Does my Child have Sensory Processing Disorder?

If your child is reacting badly to certain sounds, they are likely suffering from chronic sound sensitivity. According to the American Academy of Audiology, sensory sensitivities occur when a child becomes overstimulated by an excessive amount of one type of sensory input. They can range from a loud noise causing them to have a panic attack or light and sound sensitivity. These sensory issues may cause problems with sleep as well as affect behavior and learning abilities. How can I help my child?

The key is to find what sensory input their body is overreacting to and then either avoid it or teach your child how to cope with it.

The first step is figuring out what the trigger is and trying to find ways to overcome it. If your child has issues with sound, consider earphones or noise-canceling headphones. Next, you should keep a journal of things that may be causing the issue, such as what time they do best in school classes and at home, as well as how their body reacts to certain foods. Keep track of any progress you make in managing your reactions to stimuli.

The next step is to identify the source of the sensory input that is causing your child to react. Often, children will become more ill or be less sensitive when they are tired. They may also get less sick if they go through a period of having better hygiene habits.

If your child is overreacting to something such as cold air, then it may be beneficial for them to stay in a warm environment. Certain smells and toxins can also cause reactions in children who have sensory issues, so it's important that you find out what triggers their sensitivities.

It's crucial that you keep a detailed journal of how your child reacts to certain stimulants, as well as how often they have reactive episodes with different stimulants. This can help when you're trying to determine what the source of the issue is.

The key to having your child overcome their sensory issues is to either avoid the trigger or figure out how to make your child feel comfortable around it. This requires a lot of research, as well as some trial and error before you can find something that works for your child.

If you suspect that your child may have ADHD, conduct an assessment with a professional psychologist. They will be able to determine if they have ADHD or a different disorder. They will also help you and your child learn how to deal with these issues so that they can live happy and fulfilling life.

CHAPTER 6:

Touched by the Beauty of Emotionality

Highly sensitive people are also more affected by environmental factors than others. If they are experiencing physical pain, their emotional pain will increase as a result. They have a high level of empathy and often feel the emotions of others as their own. They can easily understand how someone else might feel in the same situation or understand how another person might be feeling even when they're unable to express themselves well. They may also find it hard to say no or to speak up for themselves—especially if they aren't sure if they want something. They don't like to feel like they're neglecting the needs of others. They are also extremely conscientious and hold themselves to high standards.

Highly sensitive people value harmony in all situations and try to avoid conflict. While this trait may not always be associated with positive feelings, it has its benefits. They may be more creative and intuitive than others and able to observe things that others might miss. They are usually more empathetic than others, which makes them good at understanding and connecting with other people on a deeper level. They are often good listeners and enjoy helping others. If you feel easily overwhelmed by things like bright lights, loud noises, or big crowds, then you might be a highly sensitive person. Some of the other traits of highly sensitive people include: having very long-lasting feelings, being bothered by excessive noise or light, being more creative and intuitive than others, having a great memory, being more emotionally reactive to both positive and negative experiences in comparison to others. These traits generally occur in both men and women but are more commonly found in women.

High sensitivity, also known as sensory processing sensitivity (SPS), is a personality trait of people who have a sensitive nervous system. While there are similarities between introversion and autism, it's not the same thing, and people can be highly sensitive extroverts or highly sensitive introverts. A 2008 study found that 15-20% of the population is highly sensitive while another 25% are only somewhat so. The trait of high sensitivity was originally defined in 1995 by Elaine Aron, who wrote "The Highly Sensitive Person." She noticed that some people seem to have more sensory nerve endings than others and are therefore extremely aware of their environments. Sensitive people are more easily affected by external stimuli than others and more easily overwhelmed. Sensitivity doesn't always imply being emotionally fragile. Sensitive people may be highly emotionally balanced and be able to manage difficult emotional experiences quite well.

Research has shown that highly sensitive people are subject to adverse effects from ambient lighting, harsh sounds, or other sensory bombardments. For example, it has been demonstrated that exposure to an overly bright environment can cause changes in the biological rhythms of the brain, such as changes in melatonin secreting cells, which in turn affects sleep patterns and can bring on a range of health symptoms, including mood alterations such as irritability or depression. The different people who have this trait may have different results. For example, some highly sensitive people are less affected by auditory and tactile stimuli. They may be able to walk in a noisy room without reacting, while others find that background noise makes it hard to focus on the task at hand. Other highly sensitive people are very sensitive to heat and cold, but some find themselves cold even though they're dressed for the weather. Still, others might not have any problems with temperature changes except when exposed to extremely hot or cold temperatures for an extended period of time.

People with high sensitivity generally have heightened awareness as well as enhanced ability to understand what is going on in other people's lives. They can be highly caring and compassionate and deeply connected to others. While they are usually highly introverted, sensitive people tend to be extremely sensitive to the external environment. They are also extremely sensitive to interpersonal conflicts and may feel irritated or hurt by things such as criticism or a lack of appreciation. Given that many highly sensitive people have low levels of assertiveness skills and the ability to effectively communicate their feelings effectively (possibly due to an effortful processing style), it is not uncommon for them to be unsure of how much they should communicate with others given their own personal limits.

Highly sensitive people can have a difficult time getting out of their own heads and expressing their thoughts. They may avoid social situations or conversations that involve many people, or even if they do choose to interact, it may feel forced. They are more likely to believe that others cannot see what is going on in their heads than most other people. They tend to be worried about not being understood by others. Those with this trait often have difficulty saying no and tend to worry that they are getting in the way of others or excluding themselves from social situations.

"The Highly Sensitive Person" is a book written by Elaine Aron that explains the traits associated with highly sensitive people. High sensitivity (SPS) is not the same thing as introversion, although many highly sensitive people do exhibit some of the characteristics of introverts. Highly sensitive extroverts are just that—high-sensitivity extroverts who are able to withstand extreme and unattractive circumstances. Highly sensitive extroverts feel energized by being surrounded by people, but they can also have other physical or mental health problems related to their sensitivity. Those who have a high degree of this trait often use social skills development techniques and/or learn coping strategies in order to function well in a social setting. In her research, Aron found that highly sensitive people showed the following traits:

- Sensitive people can be more successful in careers such as fashion design, social work, artistry, music, and poetry.
- They may also function well as counselors or nurses.
- Highly sensitive people may well have gifts for writing or other artistic endeavors. Some may have other talents, such as the ability to work with people and make them feel happy. If these people are not able to express themselves, they can experience a loss of confidence.
- They may have problems with shyness and social anxiety.
- They may also suffer from extreme sensitivity to pain, heat, cold and bright lights.

If highly sensitive people are aware that their high sensitivity might cause them problems in life, they can seek psychological therapies such as neurolinguistic programming (NLP) or hypnotherapy which has been shown helpful for highly sensitive people in many different industries. Gestalt therapy could also be used to help manage the extreme anxiety or stress that is often associated with having a high degree of this trait.

CHAPTER 7:

Autism and High Sensitivity (Differences and Similarities)

The Differences Between High Sensitivity and Autism

If you've ever been told that you are too sensitive or have taken a test for which one of the categories is too much concern for others, you might be wondering if you might actually have high sensitivity. This is an issue with many similarities to autism. One of the main differences is that many, if not most, highly sensitive people (HSPs) are sensitive because they're very happy in different degrees to all other categories on the Sensitivity Index. They enjoy themselves more in life than average, it seems. The average HSP will be a generalist. This means that they can do most things but may not be particularly good at any of them. (Most people aren't.) It also means that HSPs are more likely to savor the little things in life and to have a strong aesthetic sense.

Highly sensitive people tend to be more introverted than most. They may enjoy their own company very much and/or find it hard to socialize with others in groups and tolerate large amounts of noise or commotion. Friendships are often deep and long-lasting. They can be very sensitive to their own emotions, especially in childhood. They may dislike someone very much and still want to spend time with them. They might not like the sound of their own voice and find it hard to hear themselves speak or have conversations. They are more likely than average to have experienced trauma, especially emotional trauma, in childhood. They can also be more sensitive than average when experiencing others' emotions, even though they may not understand why other people feel the way they do about certain situations (especially if it is an overwhelming emotion).

High sensitivity isn't a disorder or a sign of low self-esteem or mental illness. It's just a natural sign of being highly sensitive that some people are more sensitive to than others. Many people in the general population are very sensitive to others. They will feel emotion with other people and notice other people's emotional states. The HSP, however, may have a greater capacity to be affected by those emotions in others than most. This could be physically sensitive such as physical complaints related to emotional distress or stress. It could also be emotionally sensitive such as tears or sadness.

The HSP may find that they don't need to make up their own stories about what is going on with other people because it is so clear in their environment. They just know that everyone is upset or unhappy about something, and they can relate on an almost unconscious level. It can also be very easy for them to read the emotions of others and to pick up on other people's emotional states. They are able to understand other people far more easily and read their emotional states than is considered normal. They will find it easy to get upset by what other people do, which other people will find difficult to understand. For example, the HSP might cry because they want others to be happy or smile when they don’t feel like it. They may really care about someone and find that they cannot stop thinking about them even though they're not with them anymore.

Highly sensitive people often have a large capacity for empathy. They may empathize with strangers more than most people would. This can lead to them feeling distressed by the world and wanting to make a difference by helping others or doing something about it. It may mean that they find it easy to read other people's emotions and body language, and as such, they are good at picking up on lies. It is very likely that they can tell if someone is lying even if they don’t know why, but this will be different for every individual highly sensitive person.

Many of them have a keen sense of smell and strong senses in general. They may hate loud sounds or prefer peace and quiet so others cannot hear them think. Their senses will often be very acute. They can feel the world around them much more easily and will often find any changes in their environment very disturbing. Every highly sensitive person is different, and sensitivity is not the same for everyone. You may be extremely sensitive to loud noise such as a rock concert or a vacuum cleaner, but not at all to other things like people who constantly use the words 'I' and 'me.'

Some people may be more emotionally sensitive than others. They might experience great distress over small events or have a sense of hyper-awareness of other people's emotions. They may find that they want to avoid offending people or that they worry about other people's feelings a lot, or simply don't know how to comfort another person in pain. This can be incredibly exhausting and sad for someone who is highly sensitive, but recognizing it for what it is can make all the difference.

There may be a different explanation for the anxiety and depression some highly sensitive people experience. You might have been told that you should just get over it when you've been upset or anxious because your sensitivity makes other people uncomfortable and causes you to feel sad about life in general. This is not always accurate, although it could help you understand why you feel as you do if someone points this out. You may be sensitive to the point of over-sensitivity, which can make it hard for other people to understand why you react the way you do. It is important not to punish yourself for feeling as you do because emotions are how we feel in response to our situations, and it is not always easy to control how we feel. An emotional response is much easier than trying to understand all about your situation and then trying to rationalize it—and this is exactly what most highly sensitive people will do.

It can be hard for highly sensitive people to handle big life changes. You may feel as though you are 'going crazy' when you are going through some sort of emotional upheaval. It can be especially difficult if you have a sense that no one else gets how you feel, and you aren't able to do anything about it. We are all different, and reacting to different situations in a variety of ways just shows this. No matter how much someone else tries to understand, they may not be able to. They may not be highly sensitive themselves, or they might just react differently or have a different mindset than yours does. This is okay. Recommended Reading: 3 Ways to Be a Highly Sensitive Person.

Highly sensitive children are often nervous or quiet in social situations, but they can be intensely creative and artistic. Highly creative people, in general, tend to be more highly sensitive. "You can't live life half-mad." Oscar Wilde.

This is something that William Wordsworth had to face over and over again throughout his life—he was a poet! Of course, when you are highly sensitive, you may have more feelings than others, so it is important not to cut yourself down about it. If someone says you are crazy or irrational, then just remember that you may be seeing things from a different perspective. You are allowed to feel whatever you feel and to react however you need to.

Many highly sensitive people are creative, artistic, or even sensitive to the point of being psychic. If you have a highly creative or artistic personality but feel as though nothing ever works out for you, then it is important to remember that this is not your fault—it is just a part of who you are. You may be in a situation where no one else understands what you are going through, and this can cause stress and confusion; however, if it doesn't bother other people, then it really isn't that big of an issue in the scheme of life. Overheating can be made worse by being highly sensitive—but we all overheat sometimes.

There are many different types of highly sensitive people—these are some of the most common:

- **Highly sensitive artistic people**. These highly sensitive individuals usually have creative thoughts, which can lead to anxiety, very high levels of stress, and withdrawal symptoms. Normally these individuals have good problem-solving abilities and can use their creativity to find alternatives and solutions to difficulties—but this is not always the case. Highly sensitive people who do not know how to manage their energy or emotions can feel overwhelmed by everyday life and may become more emotional than others around them.
- **Highly sensitive, introspective people.** These highly sensitive individuals are more likely to withdraw from social situations because of their need for peace, quiet, and solitude in order to recharge. These people find it difficult to express what they are thinking and feeling most of the time, so they often have a feeling of isolation and not being able to

communicate how they feel—this can lead to frustration, anxiety, depression, or anger.

How to Deal with Anger Issues

So before you let things spiral out of control, it's important to take a step back and find ways to deal with anger issues. Simply put, the way you deal with your anger will determine the length of time it lasts. This is why understanding how to get rid of anger issues is important. The following tips can help you curb your aggressive impulses and get your life back on track, once and for all:

1. Know your real reasons when you get angry and respond appropriately. Many of us misunderstand what "getting angry" means in real-time situations. It is important that you know what you're reacting to and why, so you can respond appropriately.
2. Learn how to handle intense emotions. It is important that you learn how to deal with intense emotions like anger or frustration in a healthy way. This means learning how to communicate effectively and developing the ability to think rationally in times of stress or irritation.
3. Recognize when you are getting aggressive or harsh with others, not just yourself. When we become aggressive or harsh with others, we are displaying unmanageable anger issues inside ourselves—but recognizing these tendencies in yourself makes it easier to recognize them in others and adapt the appropriate responses accordingly.
4. Try to be kind to yourself when you are angry. On the flip side, when you're feeling kind to yourself as a result of anger management, it is easier for you to behave in productive and kind ways toward others.
5. Learn how to direct your energy toward important goals and projects. This means that rather than allowing anger issues to consume your life and distract you from important tasks, it is easier for you to focus on making progress toward your goals and objectives.
6. Know when you are not in control of your emotions and moods—and learn when to call someone for help. It is always valuable to know when you are not in control of your

emotions and moods. When this happens, it can be helpful to consult a therapist or counselor for assistance.

7. Learn to accept that you get angry and use that information to improve your attitude and life situation. Only by accepting that you get angry and using that information effectively can you improve your attitude and life situation over time.
8. Find ways to vent chatter—but don't do it in public places or with people who you don't know well enough to feel confident about it. It is important that you find a way to vent chatter so it does not build up inside of you. But, you must be careful about venting your anger toward strangers or in public places because it could create unnecessary conflict and issues for yourself.
9. Learn to recognize underlying emotions that make you feel aggressive, so you can handle them in a healthy way. By learning how to recognize underlying emotions that make you feel angry or frustrated, it is easier for you to handle them in a healthy way—especially when they occur unexpectedly and without warning.
10. Find ways to calm yourself down or take care of your body when you are upset with yourself or others. When you are upset with yourself or others, it is important that you find ways to calm yourself down as quickly and effectively as possible. This means learning how to peacefully calm your body and mind when necessary, using relaxation or breathing techniques.

The Similarities Between High Sensitivity and Autism

Autism and high sensitivities have many similarities. Both are thought to be genetic, both are characterized by abnormal brain growth, and both are marked by different ways of thinking. While all people with autism share the same narrow band of symptoms, people with high sensitivity often exhibit an expanded range of reactions which can include sensory hypersensitivity (to vision or sound), mood swings, a low threshold for frustration, and anxiety-fueled meltdowns. Some experts in autism research believe that many people with ASD also have sensory processing difficulties, which may make them more likely to become irritable in response to a wider variety of stimuli than someone who is neurotypical.

High sensitivity can be thought of as a continuum and not a separate diagnosis. Some research has indicated that high sensitivity differs from autism in how it manifests itself in different people. Some researchers find that people with high sensitivity tend to have a stronger reaction to sights, sounds, and textures, whereas people with autism often have stronger reactions to "thoughts" or "perceptions." This may explain how a person can become distressed over something that others around them might not even notice at all.

There are many similarities between high sensitivities and Asperger's Syndrome. High sensitivities are common among those who have been diagnosed with Asperger's Syndrome, but the difference between the two conditions is not well understood. Dyslexia and high sensitivity are often diagnosed together, although they are not the same. High sensitivity may be an example of "Asperger" syndrome. An estimated 30% to 50% of children with autism also have high sensitivity. It is theorized that this condition may have some genetic component, although the idea has remained controversial. However, it has been known for many years that individuals who are highly sensitive tend to be more likely to have an autism spectrum diagnosis than those who are not and that those who are highly sensitive tend to be diagnosed as having autism earlier in life.

There is much diversity in the way that high sensitivity manifests itself. Some highly sensitive individuals are very individualistic and are not very socially oriented. They may be sensitive to light, sound, and touch, while others may be hypersensitive only to certain foods or textures or even smells (such as those with a peanut allergy). Others are hypersensitive to sound. This may serve as a barometer for when one is anxious or upset—one will become so distressed over a loud or noisy environment that they want to leave. At the same time, another person with high sensitivity may need to keep their room very quiet at all times in order to function well. The reasoning behind why some individuals with ASD have high sensitivity is still unclear. There is no clear reason for why the symptoms seem to exist, and researchers have yet to figure out just why.

Researchers have also studied a genetic link between autism and high sensitivity but have yet to determine if there is any connection between genetics and ASD with sensory integration difficulties. In terms of treatment, all persons with autism will benefit from support in overcoming anxiety by learning what triggers it when faced with overwhelming stimuli or situations. Many people with autism also benefit from learning coping strategies that build coping skills while managing the anxiety that triggers them. Some children who are highly sensitive may require help building up their social skills. Schools that have a concern for high sensitivity need to provide a curriculum that focuses on their specific needs as well as their reasoning processes, and sensitive children need accommodations on a case-by-case basis. A psychotherapist can help a person with high sensitivity to learn how to deal with the sensitivity and incorporate coping skills that are more productive. A psychologist or psychiatrist may prescribe medication for symptoms such as auditory over-responsivity or other issues which interfere with one's daily functioning.

PART II

CHAPTER 8:

Six Ways to Help Your Sensitive Child Respond More Successfully

1. Respect your sensitive child's feelings

Ask them about their emotional needs.

Recognize that they are more socially attuned than others. Help them develop the necessary skills to respond to negative people. Educate yourself and the adults in their lives on how to meet a sensitive child's needs, including special ways of teaching and dealing with bullying behavior. Teach family members not to give advice or lectures on how your child should act but rather offer support and reassurance as they go about learning new social skills and strategies for coping with challenges. Participate in social events with your child, so he or she can see different ways of handling situations that make them anxious, hurtful, or uncomfortable.

2. Give your child control over overreactions

Early on, asking your child what they think will make them feel better when they are upset. This will help teach them to problem solve and also show you that you take their needs into account.

3. Point out the "wrong look."

The best way to help your sensitive child is to not react when they have a meltdown in public places. Let them know they can count on you to be there for them at home. If you are at the grocery store and they see something that sets them off, don't be alarmed if your child has a tantrum. Point out the "wrong look" or non-accepting stare from another adult as being the reason why it happened, as opposed to any part of who your child is, and reassure them that it's not about them.

Identify triggers for meltdowns and prepare responses in advance so you are better able to protect yourself (and others) from reactions that may be inappropriate or harmful.

4. Suggest replacement actions

- Use a gentle touch and a reassuring voice
- Teach your child that they can always say no; for example, if someone is trying to touch them when they don't want to be touched, tell them it's okay if they pull away or walk away.
- Connect with your child by using body language that shows you're listening (e.g., nodding, leaning toward your child, holding eye contact).
- Let your child know when you can't help them by telling them, "I'm sorry I can't do that right now because ____." for example, "I'm sorry I can't help you now because we are in the middle of something. Let's talk after our meeting."
- Tell your child that they can always tell you when they need help. Encourage them to ask for help when they need it.
- Let your child know that you will try to help them in a specific way when they ask for help. For example, if your child asks for help writing a report, tell them you will try to give them some feedback by asking questions.
- Let your children know that you may not be able to do everything they want or need you to do.
- Help your child feel like their opinion matters while still respecting your own opinions and beliefs. For example, say, "I think we should look at this..." or "I think I would like..."
- Provide opportunities for special interests by encouraging outside interests and activities from the beginning (e.g., provide toy workshop sessions, crafting, reading groups).
- Let your children know that you think they can do it and that you believe in them.
- Create a sense of predictability and routine (e.g., by sticking to a daily schedule).
- Let them know what to expect by warning them before changing activities. For example, say, "we are going to start the

meeting in 10 minutes" or "I'm about to turn off the TV because we need to get ready for bed."

- Learn about the different ways your child learns best so that you can better respond when they need help or want something. For example, some children learn better when they use their sense of touch or are hands-on; others may learn better when they can see visual representations (e.g., using a picture instead of writing).
- Encourage your child to play with the same toys and use the same materials as you.
- Let your child know from the beginning that you will respect their choices but that you will still be present even if they don't want your help. For example, "I'll try to be quiet if we are working on something that doesn't interest me, but I'll still be there."
- Show interest in what your child is interested in and let them know you are interested in what they do or have done. For example, say, "You must really like gardening because you've been working on it all afternoon. What else do you like to garden?"
- Accept your child's opinion; don't tell them they are wrong.
- Let your children express their feelings and reactions. Trying to stop a child from expressing how they feel will not help them learn how to control their reactions.

5. Practice different tones of voice

Talk about how you might say the same thing with different levels of energy, for example. Playing or doing fun activities with your child may help them feel more comfortable around others. When your child feels uncomfortable in a social situation, try to be a "partner" instead of a "parent." Think about how you can make activities more interactive for someone who is sensitive and introverted, like your son or daughter.

6. Teach your child a "so what?" look

Head off other children's teasing by teaching your child a "so what?" look. A "so what?" look can be one of our first reactions to things that bother or embarrass us and is often used as a way to avoid conflict. Of course, the problem with this is that, over time, it leads people to an automatic and thoughtless response when they are faced with being bothered or embarrassed. I find this article helpful in understanding how we can respond more successfully.

CHAPTER 9:

Eight Things to Say Instead of "Stop Crying"

1. Crying is ok

It's a very healthy and necessary way for children to express their feelings, and we don't need to make them stop. But sometimes, it's really difficult for grown-ups to keep from saying those three words. After all, "Stop Crying" might be the only thing a caregiver can think of when they're feeling panicked and helpless in the face of a crying child.

2. Crying is always appropriate

Whatever your child is upset about is valid. You're not crying because you're a baby. You're crying because it's hard to be a kid, sometimes. Crying is always appropriate. Whatever your child is upset about is valid. You're not crying because you're a baby. You're crying because it's hard to be a kid, sometimes.

3. Don't distract

Focus on the child and their feelings. "What happened?" "How can I help?" Ask for clarification and understanding of the child's perspective. Allow time for a response. Listening is more difficult than talking—your response may be "I don't know what to say," or you might repeat back what the child said in order to understand them better, but that doesn't mean you are not listening to them or that they're not being heard.

Tell them how you feel hearing their story, which will show that they are heard and understood: "You sound very frustrated." "It sounds like such a hard situation." You might also empathize with their experience by saying, "The way you feel makes sense because...," or, "You must be frustrated because...," or, by making a comparison with your own experience such as, "I'm so frustrated when..."

4. Don't Punish, Encourage

It's understandable to be frustrated when someone is making a mess, but the best thing you can do for them is to help them feel less bad about what they're going through. Instead of telling that person to "stop crying" or "cheer up," try saying something like this:

- It sounds like you have a lot going on. Is there anything I can do?
- I'm sorry this happened and that it made you feel really uncomfortable/upset/bad. Is there anything I can do to help?
- I've been there before, and things are hard, but you'll feel better in a bit.

What I'm trying to say is that when someone is in a bad/upsetting/irritating situation, it's normal for them to feel super miserable, and most people find their own way out. You should just let them know that you're there for them, whether they want you to or not. It's important because showing compassion means you're showing someone that they're not alone in this situation; it gives them the confidence to get their stuff together and take care of themselves in the future.

And as for the situation in question, it sounds like it's all because of a bad day, but that doesn't mean it can't be fixed or that they can't get over it. You're just trying to help them take control of their emotions and move on. Don't beat them over the head with it or tell them how they feel (because really, you don't know how they feel, and no one does!). Just be supportive and helpful because that's what your friends are there for.

That being said...

"It's true that you can never predict when your old life will catch up with you, but what you can do is make sure your life has meaning. If you fall and feel sorry for yourself, don't let your friends pick you up or encourage you to get back up. Your friends will always be there to help you make things better."

5. No, but's

I will not tolerate your tears, your sadness, or anguish. Today is a new day; tomorrow will be better. You have done this many times before, and you won't break today. Let's get back on track because I know you can do it! Yes, I'm sad, but this always passes like a storm in the desert. I'll be fine. I feel overwhelmed, but I know everything will work out fine in the end. Let's talk about it. If you're sad, tell me why you are sad, and we can work it out together! *Hugs* You're crying because of *X event*? It is not the end of the world, and you can deal with this without needing to be miserable about it. Are you worried about *X event*? Let me reassure you that everything will be ok. I know we have to get to work, but today is a rest day. No one cares if we are busy, so I'm not working on this right now. We can catch up tomorrow when you are ready! I'm sure we can come up with something more useful than 'stop crying'.... *Hugs*All of these are much better because instead of telling someone to stop crying (which is a manifestation of your needs), you help them to calm down or distract them with other things. If you are in a relationship, make sure you listen to their problems and don't just tell them 'stop crying,' but actually listen to why they are sad and try to help them! Hugs always help too.

6. Ask too many questions

"Why are you crying?" "What's wrong?"

"You can't tell me what's wrong if you don't stop crying."

"Are you done now? What happened?"

7. Say, "it's ok."

Say, "I'm sorry you're upset." Say, "let me help you fix it." Say, "I can't believe this is happening to you. I know just how hard this is."

Say, do what you need to say, at the moment, for that person and for yourself. But don't say stop crying! When someone cries, we want to connect with them; we want them to know that we really get it. We want them to feel cared for and understood, not shamed or made worse by our words. The last thing they need is for us to tell them to stop crying! It can make people feel ashamed of natural response like they are being given the cold shoulder when all they needed was kindness. Stop-criers often don't know what to say, so their stop-cry comes out as a command or an insult. Saying "stop crying" is a natural reaction, but it's not the most helpful. Instead of saying 'stop crying,' try saying the opposite. Saying stop crying is like telling someone to stop feeling emotions—it's a wholly inaccurate command. Instead, you might say: I get it; this is hard; you're upset; I'm here for you; let me help carry some of this load for you. The best thing you can do for someone who's stopped crying is to hold them instead of telling them to stop. If a friend is in the middle of crying, the best thing you could do for them is put your arm around their shoulders and let them cry. This might not be what they want—they may not want to feel that way, and there are no guarantees that someone will necessarily feel comforted by your touch—but it will be much kinder than telling them to stop crying. It might seem like a small difference, but the words you say matter. If you are concerned that someone's crying may be a sign of more serious problems, it's best to suggest seeking help for that person rather than confronting them about their crying or telling them to stop. If someone is in the middle of crying, it's best not to tell them to stop. Instead, try saying, 'I get it; this is hard; you're upset; I'm here for you; let me help carry some of this load for you. Even if your friend's crying is just their way of dealing with a difficult situation, it will be much kinder to let them do it themselves.

8. Have a time limit

Sounds like you had a really tough day!

How are you feeling right now?

What would make you feel better?

Do you want me to leave so that you can be alone and cry?

Is there anything I can do to help make this better for you?

It sounds like something really tough happened. You're not weak or crazy. It's totally normal to be sad or frustrated about it. If someone wants to talk about their feelings, they will bring it up themselves, stop crying in the meantime, and then have a conversation with that person when they're ready. One of the worst things anyone can say is "stop crying," which often makes the person start crying again out of anger.

CHAPTER 10:

Tips to Help Your Child with that Mental Edge

1. Acquire basic skills

Teach kids how to navigate basic skills, such as learning to swim, riding a bike, and answering the phone. These skills will help prepare them for necessary challenges in the future.

Help them explore their interests. Encourage children to explore what they are interested in by setting up a bank account and give them an allowance each week for their efforts. This will teach kids to work hard for what they want and that time is money.

Explore teaching children to use math when shopping. As difficult as it may seem, this skill will be essential later on in life when it's time to balance a checkbook or prioritize bills for payment due dates. Teaching this skill early on will also make money management easier for kids down the road simply because they understand the importance of being financially literate at an early age.

Teach your child to save. Teach your kids the value of savings by putting money in a bank account for them.

Teach kids to earn and spend wisely. Teaching children the value of money is essential for their future success. Giving them an allowance is one way to teach them how to manage money, but giving them a chore that they must pay you hourly for is another way of encouraging children to manage their finances correctly and responsibly.

Teach kids how to be proactive with their health care needs. Whether kids have a well-child checkup, are at the dentist, or need to see a doctor, help them schedule an appointment and pay for it out of pocket. The benefit to this is that your child will learn how to be proactive when facing an illness, and they will realize the importance of healthy daily habits.

Give kids an allowance. Allowance is a great way for children to learn responsibility at an early age while also teaching them the value of money. Children should receive an allowance that they're required to save up in order to buy something special they want. This encourages kids to plan their money wisely so they can save up for big-ticket items such as a bike or computer game. Teach kids about setting goals. Whether a kid wants to earn money for an upcoming trip, save up for a special toy or put money away for a new bicycle, they have to set goals and keep track of their accomplishments. This will make it easier for them to reach their final goal while also encouraging them to never give up when they get off track.

Encourage your child's interests. If your child is interested in something, teach them how to master it at an early age by setting goals with them and giving them the freedom to explore that interest without worry that they won't accomplish something on their own. This will also teach them that they can achieve anything if they work hard to reach their end goal.

Teach kids about organizing a home business. Many households have the ability to run an efficient, home-based business. Whether it's receiving items for resale on eBay or selling homemade goods and crafts at a local farmer's market, encouraging children to explore this with you will help your child become a responsible entrepreneur down the road.

Teach your child how to tackle homework. Your child should always be doing homework, but it doesn't have to be stressful for either parent or child. If you're able to help your child organize his work time and set goals with him, homework time will be less stressful all around.

Teach kids about using a debit card. It's easy for kids to run up a bill if they misplace their spending money or don't realize how much is spent on everyday items. When your child is allowed to use a debit card, he or she will understand the importance of balancing the amount spent and staying within spending limits (such as an allowance).

2. Try something new

Do something new. Surround yourself with new people. Be curious.

Don't compare yourself to someone else. Just be who you are and do what you love.

3. Discourage complaining

Encourage creativity. Provide plenty of praise. Hold high expectations. Don't allow the child to be a victim. Teach by example. Set clear and realistic goals for your child each day, week, and month (and reward accomplishments). Allow your child to make mistakes once in a while when there are no consequences for their actions or approval is not given when they do something well. Encourage problem-solving skills with logic puzzles or games that challenge children's cognitive and reasoning abilities (such as Chess).

4. Find your voice

You never know when a child will find something they love to do. Encourage them to play with their voice and be creative by taking pictures, singing songs, or telling stories.

5. Revisit tough experiences

When your child is struggling in school, do you tell them that it's ok? That the test is so easy, and they'll do fine? While these encouragements may be true, they don't really help your child overcome their academic struggles. You have to help them see how to approach this type of challenge in the future. If your child has a tough time with math, for example, have them talk about a time they struggled with math and how they overcame that. If it's English, make sure to talk about things like recognizing language patterns or common mistakes when constructing sentences. Either way, you want to make sure that your child is reminded of the struggles they may have had and how to overcome them.

CHAPTER 11:

How Do You Deal with a Child Who Doesn't Listen

How do you deal with a child who doesn't listen? How do you deal with the frustration and anger that's been building up because you keep telling them to stop and they don't?

1. Try to figure out what is motivating the child's behavior.
2. Take a break if necessary, but don't let too much time pass before seeking out an answer.
3. Figure out what your goal is in making them listen, then devise a plan to get there effectively
4. Identify at least two or three specific strategies for each of these goals, and it may not take as long as you think!
5. Choose one strategy when it seems like the best option at the moment; try that first and see how it goes!
6. If you haven't succeeded in a while, try a different strategy. Rinse and repeat.

Perhaps this sounds simple, but it really isn't easy to keep track of all the possible situations that could occur and the consequences they would have. It's also much easier to argue with something or someone than it is to describe why they are acting a certain way.

A child who doesn't listen is not being rude. They are a kid. It's hard to be a kid sometimes, and that's okay. A child who doesn't listen is not being stubborn or childish; they are trying their best, and that's okay too.

A parent's job isn't to change the behavior of their child; it is to help them to accept the behavior of their children so that they can learn from them. If this means ignoring a misbehaving child once in a while, it may be necessary in order for them to learn how to get their way when they want something and have every reason to believe they can get it by being persistent (like when you're hungry and need food). Of course, it's okay to teach a child how to listen, but they will get "listen-trained" so much more easily when they are older and have more inhibitions about making bad choices. If something is important enough, eventually, the child is going to stop making those choices.

In order for a child to understand what their parents are saying, they need to pay attention and listen carefully. They need the tools to deal with situations when something isn't going as planned. The mother who tells her son not to swing on the monkey bars can use a stop sign or deadline (seen in this video below) as an acceptable alternative when he doesn't listen. As a parent, it is your job to help your child learn and understand what their actions mean.

Accepting and understanding the consequences of their actions is one of the most important skills that every child must learn. It can be difficult for children as they get older because they want something new, even if it means giving up something else later (and taking responsibility for both parts of this tradeoff).

The parents who would rather wait until after a birthday party to give their kids an allowance are failing the kids as support systems for learning to accept the consequences. You're doing them a disservice by ignoring this crucial skill. It's okay to offer an alternative, but you need to allow them to make the tradeoff.

Parents who would rather wait until after a party to teach their kids about decision-making are also failing the kids. They are teaching them without fully understanding how to learn best. They have an idea of how they want things done, so they create a system that is perfect for their little world. Now it's time for the child to put that knowledge into practice and make decisions on their own.

Children aren't always going to follow your instructions—at least not in all situations and with all situations you can anticipate—but there is always an alternative, even if that alternative leads them straight back into trouble.

Children who don't listen aren't being rude; they are children learning how to make decisions. They are learning that they don't always have to listen or obey because sometimes those rules just don't make sense.

Children who don't listen aren't being stubborn; they're just trying to get the most out of life. They want the most options and choices possible, and sometimes that means doing what you tell them not to do.

Children who don't listen aren't being childish; they're kids.

It's okay to feel frustrated when your child doesn't listen. It's okay to want them to listen better, but it's not their fault if you can't make them see the "right" way. He probably isn't going to stop, so what are you supposed to do? How can you help him learn how to get what he wants without violating your rules?

Until we know exactly how kids learn in order to teach them the skills they need, we'll probably continue to have a hard time figuring out how we can help them become lifelong learners and responsible adults.

A child who doesn't listen is not being rude; they're just a kid.

Do's and Don'ts When Your Kids Won't Listen

1. Don't view discipline as punishment

Discipline may feel as though you're punishing your kids. However, discipline is a necessary component of raising responsible adults. It's important to set guidelines and expectations for both yourself and your child. You should never feel the need to punish your child excessively or address every infraction, especially when they're not aggressive in their defiance.

2. Do find opportunities for praise

It's important to pay attention to what your child is doing. It doesn't do any good to point out all the wrongs and ignore the rights. Doing this will encourage your child to continue their misbehavior. Avoidance is a better solution when it's appropriate, such as taking time out for dinner or skipping chores that are too demanding of attention.

3. Do set limits and keep them

Don't let your kid get away with everything. Do give the child consequences to help them understand the difference between right and wrong. Don't hit your child or lose your temper when they are out of control. Do make sure to sit down and have a conversation with them when they're calm too, not just when they're "in trouble. Setting limits is important for kids so that they know what's okay and what's not. It helps them understand where the line is without feeling like adults are making up rules left and right, just so that they can be in charge all of the time. When a child knows what to expect, it also means more predictability in their life which brings peace for everyone involved. When your kid isn't listening to you, it's usually because they don't want to. If the child is old enough to go outside and play, for example, they have the right to choose what they do. They're also responsible for their actions, even if you like to give them a break by letting them have their way some of the time.

It's important to teach children how to manage their emotions so that they're not out of control. When kids are young, it's best to start out with something small and work up from there. It can be helpful if you can find a way for the child to succeed and be happy about it too. In a way, it's like teaching them what's right and wrong. When kids misbehave, it might be helpful to think of the major offenders, like distracting them with another activity when they're silly or not listening.

- "Don't you want to do your math homework now?" "Don't you want to listen to me? [they'll] get in trouble if they don't do what I say—removing a privilege for a certain period of time. Leave them alone if they're not following the rules. "You need to stop jumping on the couch and on other people's stuff. You can't play with your friends for the next two hours because you're getting in the way of their toys. "
- Doing a chore for a certain period of time. Make them clean up a mess if they made it, or maybe they have to sit in time out without playing too. "You need to put your toys away now so that everyone can have plenty of room to play.

- Taking away something they like and are attached to. They might not like it at first, but over time they'll begin to understand that there are consequences for their actions. "You're not going to get that picture you wanted today. You can't have it anymore. No TV for the rest of the weekend."
- If the behavior persists, make a plan of action so that you don't lose control. The child will hopefully remember what happened after they had some time to think about it and won't repeat their behavior in the future. Maybe they'll understand why they should listen better next time, or maybe you'll arrange to have them go see a therapist get some help with them getting out of control more easily and quickly.

Make sure that you have compassion for your children at all times because they're by no means perfect. When they "misbehave," it probably means that they're upset about something or feeling overwhelmed. Try not to be so judgmental about whatever is going on that you can't give them the time of day to hear what it is. It's never a good idea to punish children for their feelings of frustration and anger. Instead, teach them how to manage those feelings and talk them through everything to help get rid of the negative pressure as quickly as possible. Remind them of what the consequences are too. You shouldn't be too quick to punish because you don't want them to learn that everything's taken away from them if they're not good or that it's okay to get away with bad behavior and not feel any consequences for it. If they learn this early on, then they'll be more likely to repeat it in the future or, even worse, when they're older. The key is to make sure that there's always a consequence in place so that they won't know what else is out there for them. When everyone's calmed down and ready to listen again, sit down with your child and have a conversation about what happened. It's a great idea to speak in a calm but stern voice so that they understand your position. You don't want them to figure out how to trick you or figure out ways around the rules if they know what you're looking for.

The discussion should help them see that what they did was wrong and teach them that there are consequences for their actions. It's also important to let your child know that it wasn't just an accident or a coincidence when they misbehaved. If not, then it's going to be really hard for them to learn from their mistakes later on in life, too, once it becomes clear to them what happened.

“You weren't supposed to bite your brother because he tickled you."

"Mommy and Daddy were watching the TV, and you ran into the room without permission. You hurt yourself."

"Because of your behavior, you've lost the privilege of having more toys for a while."

As with any rule that you set forth, it's important to make sure that the child understands why it is. If they don't understand, then they might think that their actions were justified in some way after all. Of course, if you're too harsh about it, then you could end up losing them forever. The key is to make sure that they understand the rules and procedures so that they can use them later on in life when necessary. For example, if you're only allowing your child to have one cookie, then it's important that they know why. You don't want them to think that you're taking away something from them without a good reason to do it. On the other hand, if you're allowing your child to have one cookie because it's dessert time, then maybe letting them know when dessert time it will help as well. It should also be easy for them to know that they have more than one cookie whenever dessert rolls around again without having any problems. Another helpful way to get this all straight in their mind is for you to write a time-out punishment chart as part of your set of procedures. That way, they'll know exactly what they've done and how they're supposed to act if they want to use the privileges again. It will be much easier for them to understand how the rules work between each other. Still, it's important that you don't feel pressured or even threatened by your child's behavior if you're going through with this during the first few months of life.

It's better to let the child know that his or her behavior was inappropriate and that you're not going to stand for it instead. Then you can decide what best to do on your own. Always remember, it's important that you be firm and consistent with your children from the beginning. It'll make them feel more secure in themselves once they get older, and they might even learn some good lessons from this as well as needing to behave more. You'll also find that life will be much easier for both of you when you do this. In the end, you'll be glad that you stuck to your guts, or you'll regret it in the future. There's no question that starting out right from the beginning is better than having to start over after some bad behavior later on. It's best to make this easier on yourself now by choosing a time-out punishment system that works well. You might even find this to be a lifesaver in a time of need.

4. **Don't threaten or explode. It does not get better**

Don't push them to talk about what's wrong. Let them know you're there for them, instead of trying to make them feel uncomfortable with your prying questions, or worse yet, pushing their problem under the rug, so you have as little work as possible.

Do have clear and consistent rules that are followed by everyone in the family. This will help set expectations and eliminate confusion on what is and isn't appropriate behavior in any given situation.

5. **Do be a parent, not a buddy**

Encouraging your kids to spend time with you does not necessitate you directing all their activities. Don’t give in to parental guilt. Parenting is hard work, but it's not a competition or a performance of self-sacrifice. You're entitled to take care of yourself, too! Do model the behavior you want them to follow. Children learn more from observing adults than they do from instructions alone. If you want your child to practice good manners, make sure that when eating dinner together, everyone says please and thank you and occasionally asks questions about each other's day. Don’t be surprised if they don't follow your example. People learn by seeing others practice what they preach, not simply be advised to practice it. Kids are no exception.

Do good model behavior yourself—especially when you're stressed or tired or in a rush. Children are particularly perceptive about when their parents are rigid, irritable, and insensitive, and if that's the model you set for them, they'll learn to treat others poorly as well. Don’t demand respect if you haven't earned it. You can tell your children what you expect from them without demanding respect in return. You're not entitled to respect until you've earned it first. Do be consistent in the way you communicate with them. You can't tell a kid that one thing is OK one time, and then the next day says they're ridiculous for doing it. If you want your child to know why a behavior is inappropriate, explain your reasoning in as clear and straightforward manner as possible, without resorting to insults or character assassination.

6. **Don't lecture or scold or talk over them if they're talking with you**

Be patient even with kids who aren't listening. Ask questions instead of making assumptions about their thoughts or feelings. Do make eye contact. When adults look at children directly, they communicate that the child is important to them and that they're interested in what the child has to say. Don't interrupt your children when they're speaking to you. A child who's interrupting you is a problem for the parent, not the child. People can tell when you've been interrupted during a conversation: Your body language changes; your tone becomes hostile; your message becomes less clear and less complete; and your ability to listen diminishes—all signs that you've lost focus on what's really important and stopped paying attention to what someone else actually said.

7. **Do let your kids help you with chores**

Kids who learn responsibility by helping around the house and making their own bed or setting the table for dinner will not think of cleaning, setting the table, or washing dishes as chores to be avoided. Don't worry unduly about a mess. Kids' rooms will be messy until your children have a good reason to keep them neat—usually because they're their own boss, they have a job where neatness is important, or they're living in an apartment or dorm room where messes aren't tolerated. Leave your kids alone to figure out what's important and what's not on their own without stepping in to make decisions for them.

Do help your kids learn how to cook and clean. Food preparation skills are important but not as important as communication skills in the long term. Teaching your children to cook and clean will put them on the path to financial independence.

8. Don't travel long distances with kids in tow

This poses a safety risk for all involved—not just the adults but also the child being transported. Don't let them hitch rides, set off alone on foot, or use public transportation without adult supervision until they're much older and better able to handle unfamiliar situations and navigate by themselves safely.

Do encourage kids to get involved in sports or other activities that require their time, particularly if they're boys. Children who are physically more active have a lower risk of obesity and depression. Don't try to make your children popular. Focus on raising happy, healthy children—not popular ones. If you provide your children with enough time, protection, and boundaries, you don't need to worry about whether they're popular or not.

9. Do help your kids learn how to interact well with others

Instead of telling your children how to behave, teach them that everyone is different. Encourage them to be open-minded and curious about others and spend time with people who are unlike themselves, not just like them. Don't make your kids feel guilty for having a different life from the one you had growing up. You can't prepare them for what they can't possibly imagine. And remember that it's okay for their lives—and their behavior—to change as they move through adolescence!

Do encourage your teens to think independently, even if it makes you uncomfortable when they come up with an unconventional opinion or idea. Let them know you respect their intellect and individuality and are curious to hear what they have to say.

10. Don't try to change who your children are

Acceptance is the best gift you can give your children. Children look for approval from the adults in their lives, so if someone they love loves them, even with all of their flaws, they feel better about themselves out of the gate than if no one loves them at all. Be that person for your kids—always! Do offer your teens a goodnight kiss every night. It might seem silly, but a nightly ritual like this helps everyone reestablish each day's love in a way that may be forgotten in the bustle and stresses of everyday family life. Don't pressure your teens to have sex. It's not a medical issue (not at this time, anyway). Don't make your kids feel like they have to do it or that you feel obligated to have them do it. There are many other ways to stay safe and healthy—healthy relationships, healthy minds, healthy bodies, and healthy communities all need good models of love instead of sex. If they aren't going to be with the person who makes them feel safe and loved in life when they're young, there are still plenty of other people who can provide for that need later in life. Do stop dating your children's friends. This can only end badly for everyone involved, and it's not fair to try to prevent your kids from dating a certain person just so you can date them yourself. Don't check your kids' rooms all the time. Sure, you might find some things that make you uncomfortable—from their porn stash to their guns—but these are messages they're sending out about themselves. If you respond by saying what they want to hear instead of allowing them autonomy, they'll be more likely to continue to keep secrets from you in the future and engage in behaviors that are unhealthy for them.

11. Don't forbid your kids from doing things

That just makes them want to do it even more, and it can cause resentment. Instead, teach them that there are consequences for their actions no matter what they're doing—good or bad. Tell them ahead of time what those consequences will be and stick by your word; don't wiggle around on the discipline because you think it'll make yourself feel better about not wanting them to engage in a certain behavior (or because you're afraid they'll get mad at you).

Don't make it seem like you want more children. Once a couple has one child, they often assume that's enough—even though it's not. This can lead to resentment when others get pregnant, and you might even think your child might be better off in a different family.

Do ask kids about their sexual histories. The more they know about what happened to them as sexual beings, the better equipped they'll be to deal with the realities of sex in later life (such as how they're going to react when someone tries to touch them inappropriately). It also helps them understand why other people have sex and what makes some people act out sexually and others not—which is important information for any kid. The more they know about what happened to them as sexual beings, the better equipped they'll be to deal with the realities of sex in later life (such as how they're going to react when someone tries to touch them inappropriately). It also helps them understand why other people have sex and what makes some people act out sexually and others not—which is important information for any kid. Discuss how you want your child to behave sexually someday. If you know you want your child to wait until marriage to have sex, talk about that together. If you don't care if he or she ever has sex at all and are more concerned about preventing pregnancy, discuss that instead. When talking about sex with your teenager, be yourself.

Don't feel the need to impart your values to them. There's nothing worse than having a 45-minute lecture about how you were a screw-up when you were a teenager, and now you're disappointed in yourself. It's better to present the information in age-appropriate terms and then use it as an opportunity to discuss how you handled things at that age. You raised a baby, so you must have done something right!

Setting Rules

How can I work out the problems I have with my teen? I want her to respect me, but she feels like she has no rules.—Julie C. To set the groundwork for respecting you and treating you with respect, she needs to know that she has rules—and why.

Rules are necessary for any relationship, even the best of them. If there are no rules, what stops her from being impulsive and doing whatever she wants? You're going to have to lay down a few guidelines of your own so that your teen can't get by with breaking the rules you lay out—if she ever does. It's very difficult to build trust and respect in a relationship when one person feels like they have no boundaries or limits on how far they're allowed to go. If you're constantly stressed or frustrated by your teen's behavior, it can't be long before she's just going to react the same way—and that'll lead to a very uncomfortable relationship. So what do you need to do? First, be sure there are no unspoken rules in place; when you think about what your teen is doing and why she's done it, try to put yourself in her shoes. Know what she thinks makes sense; know what she believes are acceptable boundaries for her. Ask yourself which rules make sense and which ones don't. You'll probably start by laying down some general guidelines that apply to all of your interactions with her. These should be the same for everyone in the household, though, not just for your teen. Ask your teen if she agrees with them—maybe she'll suggest a few other rules that you'd both be comfortable with. The more it feels like a joint decision made by you both, the better she'll feel about her ability to respect those rules (and you) because they're something you've all agreed upon together. This is also where you can start to teach her how to communicate her needs or wants—in a way that works best for her as an individual. (If she's like most teenagers, she'll be better at communicating on social media than in person.) Make it clear to her that you're willing to listen and talk about anything anytime—as long as you're both able to remain calm. You can also let her know that if she needs help with a problem, you'll be there for her; the same goes for her friends. You might want to set up time blocks in your teen's schedule when he has nothing else going on so that he'll have more time—but not too much time—to spend with you without feeling pressured by all the other things going on during the day. (This might be something you and your spouse need to discuss, gradually increasing the number of blocks he has as he gets a little older.) But do remember that his schedule is his own—always make sure that there are no obligations or distractions (including calls or texts from friends) during these scheduled times. Your teen's first year will be full of change. She'll want to see many different friends and hang out with them when she doesn't have other commitments scheduled. Make sure your teen understands that she can still call you anytime if she needs help, but it's okay if she wants to talk to one or more of her other friends instead. Remember that she's still learning who she is, and she'll—at least at first—feel most comfortable with people who share similar interests as her. As you work together to build the kinds of rules you both want in your family, consider making some small changes now to lay a foundation for a great future relationship. (For example, consider swapping out your teen's mattress for one that's softer.) For now, this may just be about you and your spouse setting boundaries and having some rules that make sense to you both so that the rest can take care of themselves down the road.

CHAPTER 12:

Sports and Sensitive Children

Sports can be a scary time for sensitive kids. The new environment and the changes in routine can cause some to feel overwhelmed and anxious. There are many things you can offer to make this stage of your child's development easier. Below I'll discuss some tips for getting through sports with a sensitive child so that they too may enjoy the benefits of team-building and fun associated with playing on a sports team.

- Discuss what to expect before the season starts. A lot of parents underestimate how nervous their children might feel about starting an activity they haven't tried before and don't talk about it much beforehand, which is why it's important to take notes from other parents who've been there before or are currently experiencing these feelings themselves. Your child will be anxious, and it is your responsibility to prepare them for what they will be facing.
- On the first day, make a joke about being nervous and ask them about their experiences with starting new teams in the past. It'll let your child know you understand how they feel and may even help you see some similarities between you and your child.
- Be positive about their experiences on their first day. If they are too nervous to enjoy themselves, let them know that it's okay—tell them that everyone was nervous at one point in time or another and that practice will make them better at it.
- Offer to help them with their bags and equipment. It's ok if they don't want your help at first, but eventually, they will need you! They probably won't have someone to help hand them weights and balls or understand how a certain level of fit works on their shirts. If you're going to offer, it's important to be a helpful teammate.

- Bring extra clothes for your child if it's cold or rainy out. Having an extra pair of socks and extra shorts can be nice for those sudden showers that come up at practice and the rain that inevitably falls during the games, especially if they've only brought one set of clothes.
- Don't let their anxiety ruin the experience for other members of the team. While it's important to be understanding and help your child through their time of adjustment, it's also important to remember that there are other teammates and parents who are counting on you to do your part. If your child is having a hard time, have a serious talk with them about how not participating can affect others or why they should at least go out and watch the others play. If you aren't willing to face these issues head-on, your child will soon be heading for trouble when they start losing interest in their sport or in doing well during practices.
- Encourage them if they seem unhappy. It can be hard for kids to see your support when they feel like there's nothing to look forward to. Encourage them to make the best out of their situation and be a good sport.
- Teammates will ask about your child's emotions, and if you don't feel comfortable talking about it, keep quiet. Your child will ask what you think they need or what you think would help them. Take the first step in helping them through by talking about their feelings about going to sports practice or going on the field. They'll respond well to positive reinforcement and encouragement from friends they trust and are likely already looking forward to practicing with in the future.
- Help them with their school work. Nothing is more frustrating than a kid who is having a hard time doing their homework because they are constantly thinking about sports. Letting your child know that you're there to help and will remind them of what they need to do will show them you care about helping them succeed in life.
- Encourage participation on the team and in practice. Be the one person that supports your child's dreams and efforts even if it isn't their forte because they might surprise themselves by

learning something new about themselves or working harder than ever before to achieve something they never thought possible before.

- Talk to other parents on the team if the problem appears bigger than what you can handle. There are always other people to talk to about your child's interests and concerns. If you don't know where to begin, friend your child on Facebook or make friends with the parents who are there for practice and encourage them to contact you if they need help or want to talk.
- Don't think that your child hates an activity when they're really nervous. If this is their first time trying something new, it can feel a bit daunting when you're put into a new situation. It's important for parents to understand the difference between a feeling of dislike and a feeling of anxiety in order not to overreact or dismiss an opinion about an activity as not worth it when they might just need some time to adjust.
- Get your child a punching bag. If your child is being bullied or has been getting into fights at school, they might want a way to express their frustration with another person. It can be hard for children to work out their feelings about bullying if it is keeping them from doing the things they like, including sports. If they are struggling in this area, getting them a punching bag can help them achieve something when things are tough at school without resorting to violence and may even keep them from feeling the need to bully or intimidate others in order to feel powerful.
- Let them know you are there for them. Sometimes in difficult situations, a parent or guardian needs to let a teenager know that the person they are counting on to guide them through life is still there for them no matter what they do, so tell him or her what you're feeling and what your plans are for the future—whether it's to be supportive during this difficult time or even if it's just to let your child know that they can call you at any time if the going gets tough.
- Strike up a conversation about their weekend over coffee with friends. If your child is not involved in any extracurricular activities, spending quality time with them and listening to

what they have to say can offer a great opportunity to open up about their feelings and what's going on at school. If you've already built a rapport with them over the years, then you can easily start conversations about how they are doing at school or even just asking them what happened during the day.

- Use your knowledge of your child's interests to gauge their emotional state. If they are always stuck in their room listening to rock music without talking to anyone else for hours on end, then you should be able to tell that something is wrong because it's out of character for them. If they don't want to talk about their friends, hobbies, or school, then you can be sure that they are having a rough time at school and may even need your help. If you notice that this isn't the case, then you should use the same system of assessment to determine if they are in a safe environment.
- If your child is not a member of any extracurriculars at school or if they are struggling to find anyone to talk to, encourage them to join clubs and sports. This will allow them the opportunity to feel what it's like for other people their age and give them someone different to spend time with when things become tough at school. If your child is a member of any clubs or sports teams, then ask them about how they feel about their team and if they are in good hands. If they are, then that means everything's going according to plan, and the reason for your concern is actually unrelated to the school.
- Remind your child that no matter how bad things get, you will always be there for them. Parents and their children are very close, and your child knows that you will always be there for them. When they feel as though they need it most, the support and encouragement from their parents can make all the difference. What is already known about this topic?

CHAPTER 13:

Bullying and Sensitive Children

Peer pressure can have a negative impact on self-esteem in schoolchildren. School bullying is an under-reported problem, with students often making excuses for their behavior or refusing to report it due to embarrassment or fear of 'getting into trouble.' There is also a lack of research into how to prevent peer victimization. Bullying at school can affect many areas of a child's life, including academic work, social relationships, and mental health issues. What does this study add? This study aimed to explore the relationship between child parenting style and peer victimization in primary school-aged children.

Parenting style (method of negotiating with a child) was measured using a short parent report form, which described infants' sensitivity, life expectancy, and autonomy agreements with their parents. This was compared to the circumstances experienced by their two best friends (the 'friends group'). The 'friends group' was also measured using a short self-report questionnaire, which collected data on bullying frequency, bullying involvement, and bullying involvement-related stress. The sample consisted of 256 children attending one primary school in Devon over an eight-week period. This was to allow a comparison of reading performance in peer groups at the same age. In a second study, 5-year-old children were assessed in 4 different social classes (half-born into the working class and half into the middle class), and results showed that there was no substantial difference between them either as regards their general levels of achievement, or their reading scores

1. These findings are consistent with other studies, which also indicate that the two classes have approximately equal levels of overall literacy and numeracy amongst children.
2. The main point to emerge from this research is that it is not easy to establish just how much we can attribute to the effects

> of peer group influence on achievement. Firstly, it is hard to find out how much any particular child is influenced by their peer group. To the extent that this is attributable to the quality of teaching in primary schools (rather than to family background factors), it may well be because primary teachers have much more contact with children than secondary teachers have.

Nowadays, I just talk about my dreams with them and tell them how it feels when you achieve something you've wanted for a very long time. They understand and sometimes even encourage me to go on adventures every day, which makes me feel like there's nothing wrong with the world or life at all. I wake up every morning feeling more determined than the last. Like many of my friends, I've had a lot of trouble with self-confidence over the years. My days of dreaming are long gone, although luckily, not so far that I can't remember everything about them. When I'm anxious or nervous about something, I think about how small and insignificant those emotions are compared to things like flying to distant planets and exploring new lands in unknown spaceships. As silly as it may sound, I feel like those kinds of dreams are more realistic than figuring out what I want to do with my life and achieving it. The thought of suicide has crossed my mind many times over the years, and I think about it every day. Some days are harder than others, and I worry that one day, it will be too hard to get through another day without giving in to the dark creatures inside my head that tell me pain is all there is.

However, usually, something good happens in my life at least once a week, and if not, then at least one person tells me something nice or does something kind for me. My school is a place where you can go to study if you want to, but it's mostly for kids who like quiet places in the morning so that they can study before class. Sometimes I wish I had more friends, but sometimes it's okay just being alone at home or with my father. My dad has been my best friend since I was very little, and anytime someone tries to bully me or someone else, he tells them that they are stupid and that no one really cares what they think about them. It makes me feel safe like I'm under some kind of protection that keeps my bad feelings away. When I was a bit younger, I used to have a lot of problems in school. Some kids would laugh at the way I talked and made fun of me because my voice sounded funny, and they'd make fun of the type of clothes that I wore, but the teachers didn't do anything about it. They'd just tell them to stop, but they never did, and it really hurt me a lot. When my parents found out what was happening at school, they called up the principal and told him they wanted him to put an end to it or else there would be consequences for him.

After that, I never heard from anyone else who made fun of me. I'm also really glad that my family and friends have been really supportive of me when it comes to making decisions about my life. I don't know what I'd do without them.

I hope someday maybe I'll have a girlfriend who would support me the way they all do, and then we can share our dreams together, the ones you make every day when you're four years old and have no idea how far away they are from reaching.

CHAPTER 14:

Highly Sensitive Child and School

If you have a highly sensitive child, it can be difficult to know how to best support them in school. Working with the school staff and providing explanations about the way your child learns can help ease their stress. We have a number of high-sensitivity resources here for parents and teachers: http://www.hsperson.com/essentials-for-parents/.

Empowering others with knowledge is an important endeavor, so we've assembled these resources on understanding highly sensitive children, teaching kids coping skills for managing their sensitivities at school, and also understanding what is considered normal emotional reactivity for kids based on our research into emotional intelligence. Our Super Sensitive Child is a great book written by an occupational therapist for parents of Highly Sensitive Children. A highly sensitive child can be very intelligent, but difficulties in school can make it harder for them to express their true intelligence. Super Sensitive Child teaches parents how to support their child at home and in school so that they can learn as much as possible. This article presents a framework based on the Tucker et al. (1990) model of emotional intelligence and provides guidelines for teaching emotional literacy in small classes. Emotional literacy involves helping students understand emotional expressions, verbal communication, feelings, and human development by providing explanations of developmental stages through which students may go.

There are many studies that research the effects of assessing emotional intelligence on student outcomes. For example, Zedeck et al. (2009), in a study examining the impact of classroom assessments on student achievement and teacher satisfaction, found that teacher ratings of students' out-come were significantly higher when students were assessed with an emotional intelligence inventory. In addition to the positive effects of emotional literacy on classroom behaviors, the benefits of teaching this type of material are significant for helping students understand their emotions and develop strategies for managing them. This article examines the affirmative action process and evaluates its potential benefits in supporting the inclusion of underrepresented groups in institutions of higher education.

Highly Sensitive Children and Highly Sensitive People

HSP/Sensory Processing Sensitivity (SPS) is a term created by Elaine Aron and Adam Bricker to describe a subset of the population who tend to be more sensitive to sensory stimulation and thus have a different experience of life such as being more easily overwhelmed. Sensitive people have nervous systems that are highly attuned to subtle stimuli. These stimuli can be anything from light, sound, smell, touch, or any combination of the five senses. There is growing evidence using multivariate statistics that HSPs and SPS people show differences in brain structure and activity during cognitive tasks. Their brains show greater activity in the right striatum (a region of the brain associated with emotion and reward) on a task that measures response to reward, while in SPS groups, we see more activity in the right insula, which correlates with higher cognitive activity and cortical attentional processes.

There is another group of highly sensitive people called "Highly Sensory Processing (HS) People," who tend to be very aware of or acutely aware of senses and their various effects. They are often good at picking up subtle changes in their environment and can become irritated or upset if things around them aren't just what they call "right." This type of sensitivity is, however, similar to what some people call "extreme sensory" or "problematic" sensitivity. Highly sensitive people and highly sensitive children are not the same things. Highly sensitive people can experience many of the same sensitivities as HSPs but also experience their sensitivities in differing ways. In fact, it is the way they are affected by these sensitivities that distinguish highly sensitive people from highly sensitive children. For example, highly sensitive children may not be very aware of their environment with regard to sensory stimulation. They may only notice if there is a commotion or disruption in their classroom environment and become very upset if the room temperature changes. Highly sensitive people, however, are more aware of their environment and are more likely to be upset if their classroom environment doesn't match the way it is "supposed" to be. The difference in sensitivity is due to what researchers call "sensory gating" or the "passive filtering" that sensitive people and children have during an encounter with sensory input.

Sensitive people and children filter out sensory information before it can affect their mood and feelings. For example, highly sensitive children may not be aware of changes in temperature or the sounds around them until they become aware that you have noticed them. Highly sensitive adults also tend to filter out negative stimuli before they cause anxiety or other effects on their mood or emotions.

Children and adults with HSC typically have a good sense of the here and now and of their sensitivities. They can experience sensations without overreacting. For example, a child who is sensitive to the smell of perfume might notice it at an appropriate level, where it doesn't interfere with their learning or social development. They would be more likely to put perfume on later if they didn't like the smell, but they would not believe that anyone else disliked it. Highly sensitive people (HSP's), however, are prone to overreacting to certain sensations. They may become overwhelmed by sensory input and become intent upon being protected from sensory intrusions.

Highly Sensitive Children (HSC's) do not know how they feel, and therefore can't tell others about their sensitivities. They may not be able to identify the source of their discomfort or inability to participate in an activity because they don't understand why it happens. Highly Sensitive People, however, are aware of their sensitivity and know how they feel when it is disrupted by new stimuli. They may be more aware of both their own needs and the needs of others.

Highly Sensitive Children can also have heightened sensitivity to everything. They are over-responsive to external stimuli and cannot tolerate loud noises, bright lights, fast movements, and other similar experiences. HSP's are also very sensitive to certain smells, tastes, and textures. These sensitivities can intensify as a child gets older—especially when they start to develop their own preferences, likes, and dislikes which can differ from those of their parents.

HSP's tend not to share their sensitivities with others unless they feel a need to do so because they feel misunderstood or stigmatized because of them. HSC's, however, often don't realize that they are different from their peers. If others experience things the same way they do, then their reactions to external stimuli must be the "right" way.

HSP's and HSC's can often benefit from a sensory diet: It is important for parents and teachers to understand that sensitivity—both in children and adults—is not about what the S stands for; it's about how sensitive people react to external stimuli—whether it is a hormone that makes them more reactive or just their normal way of living life.

How is it possible to tell the difference between an HSC and an HSP?

HSCs have one or more of the following symptoms: they are frightened by loud noises (especially unexpected ones); they are frightened by fast or jerky movements; or they startle easily; they react strongly to certain smells; they may be bothered by food tastes, textures, clothing fabrics, cosmetics, or other things in their environment; or they may feel that certain places are "wrong" due to their associations with unpleasant memories. Sweet smells often irritate them (but this can also be a sign of a medical condition).HSPs, on the other hand, are not so bothered by these things. Such stimuli might irritate them, but they can usually tolerate them. They are not frightened easily (though they may be startled or taken aback by something unexpected). But HSC's have an extremely low tolerance for anything that startles or frightens them. In addition to this wide range of sensitivities, HSC's generally do not like reading and writing. Their eyes tend to wander rather than focus on the material; their writing is messy and hard to read. They also have a hard time being patient. HSC's, on the other hand, tend to be good students and like to read and write. HSPs are often interested in a variety of subjects, especially ones that are intellectually stimulating. They enjoy working with ideas rather than things (though they have no trouble focusing on practical activities when the need arises).

- HSC's are generally much less interested in abstract ideas or intellectual discussions; they want their activities to have an immediate practical result.
- HSPs tend toward introversion; HSC's toward extraversion. Again, this is not absolute but a tendency.

- HSPs, as the name implies, are sensitive to stimuli in their environment and can be easily distracted. HSC's are more comfortable being active participants in life and may quite like having lots of stimuli.
- HSPs are generally creative and perceptive, thinking about how things should be rather than how they are; HSC's tend toward realism. Of course, there are plenty of exceptions to these tendencies.
- Many HSC's have a strong appreciation of beauty in the natural world or in music or art; many HSPs might have a great deal of psychological insight into the motivations and behavior of others. But both groups are less interested in the traits of other people than are non-sensitive people.
- HSPs are generally more sensitive to pain, smells, and tastes (e.g., they notice when things "taste funny" or "smell bad").
- HSC's have a low threshold for pain; the slightest cut or bruise can cause extreme discomfort. They tend to fear injury, especially anything that would result in blood loss. HSP's are not as aware of small discomforts, but when they do experience them, it is usually something that has been causing them concern for some time, and their reaction may be large.
- HSPs can become upset with a lack of respect, even if the actions are unconscious. HSC's are generally not bothered by such things; they may even see it as a sign of weakness in others (because someone who should be strong is not).
- HSP's can become easily overwhelmed by sensory overload; HSC's only react to it if it is too much. They have little sensitivity to touch and will welcome an opportunity to rest. Usually, they are much more responsive to changes in their environment than HSPs and don't need to be exposed to as much sensory input in order for them to become upset.
- HSP's generally have more tolerance for temperature variations than do HSC's. HSP's tend to live a more even-tempered life when it comes to temperature variations, such as keeping their rooms at a very comfortable level. HSC's may become upset if the temperature rises or falls too much.
- HSP's can react strongly to stress; HSC's can't become overwhelmed by stress and, if they do, it is usually only for a

short time. If HSP's are stressed or when they're tired but need to be "on" or don't want anything to get in the way of doing their work, they may become easily upset over small things that others would not notice. HSC's, however, are not as affected by stress and may even be able to tolerate it if they have time to decompress.

- HSP's are more likely to become upset if they have too much on their minds that they can't sort out.
- HSC's may become significantly disturbed by a change in their routines but are usually much less bothered by things that are new and unexpected. They often will not notice when a small change occurs in their environment until it becomes a big problem for them.
- HSP's are more likely to be mistaken for Asperger's syndrome. In fact, some researchers think that HSP is a much milder form of Asperger's and may even be one of the traits that people with Asperger's have in common. HSPs, on the other hand, are not good candidates for a diagnosis of AS because they have sufficient social skills (unlike children with Asperger's).
- Highly Sensitive Children often need to be encouraged to become independent. They need to be allowed to embrace their uniqueness, a quality that is special not only to them but also to others. They may know what they want but still need encouragement from others to actually go out and get it.
- Highly Sensitive Children have an exceptionally hard time learning how to socialize because they can immediately sense if others are upset or not happy with them and then become the cause of the disturbance. HSP's, on the other hand, are more comfortable with socializing if they know other people have no idea that they have sensitivity and everyone is just acting normally around them.

In order to understand the personality of an HSC, it is important to understand how they perceive and process experience. For example, if you tell them that they smell bad or are not wearing enough deodorant, they will become upset because it interferes with their ability to function in social situations. They may even feel alone in their sensitivity and not know what "normal" is. It is important to recognize that for HSC's there is no "normal" way for everyone else to act—their own method of coping with the world could be different from someone else's. It is important for parents and teachers alike to help them to become interested in new things. This is the best way to help them develop and tolerate the differences that exist between people. The more they can get out of their own head and see how other people feel, the better it will be for them.

Highly Sensitive Children tend to be very responsive both to their own needs and the needs of others. They are often more sensitive in this way than adults, who may have unconsciously developed techniques for dampening or ignoring others' needs. They need to be allowed to explore and develop their own interests, even if it does not seem to be practical at the time. They need to be given the freedom and support for this natural process. They are much more likely than HSP's to become overwhelmed by their own needs as well as those of others.

Highly Sensitive Children have a hard time saying no when someone asks them for something or demands something from them, so they need adults who will stand up for them in these situations. When an HSC is upset by a situation and doesn't know what to do about it, an adult needs to help them sort out their feelings and help them cope with whatever is upsetting them. When an HSC becomes upset, they often need time to figure out what is happening and how they feel about it.

HSP's often need more space to work on their own projects. They are more likely to see something they've wanted for a long time and take the initiative to get it than are HSC's, who may feel that someone else is holding them back or getting in the way by not providing them with everything that they want.

HSC often have a hard time in social situations; they may not be able to cope well under stress or when others make demands on them. HSP's may have difficulty communicating their needs or feelings to others. They need an adult who can help them to be able to sort out what they want and need.

If you are the parent of a highly sensitive child, then it is important that you understand how they process information and how this can affect their ability to function in the world. It is also important for you and your child to develop your own understanding of what is normal for a highly sensitive kid. Any attempt by either of you to impose on the other may lead to conflict, which would do neither of you any good. If you are a teacher of children, it is important that you understand that highly sensitive kids see things differently from the way non-sensitive kids do and therefore need different kinds of help in order to succeed academically. You may need to develop new methods of teaching for them. It is also important that you encourage them to work at their own pace and try not to push them too much.

If you are a relative or friend of an HSC, it is important that you be supportive of her interests and needs. You can provide some support by helping them to make decisions and by not making demands. If you are very close to someone who is highly sensitive, then it is especially important that you don't make demands on them as they may become overwhelmed at the thought of all the things they need to do for others. If you are an HSC, then it is especially important that you do not try to act like non-sensitive people. You need to find your own way so that others can accept your differences. It is very important to be liked by other people. You also need to feel important and valuable. It is also helpful if you can find a way to spend time alone without feeling guilty about it since HSC's are often very close to their friends and relatives. They may need someone to help them learn how to deal with stress better.

Highly sensitive children tend to be very responsive both to their own needs and the needs of others. They are often more sensitive in this way than adults, who may have unconsciously developed techniques for dampening or ignoring others' needs. They need to be allowed to explore and develop their own interests, even if it does not seem practical at the time. They need to be given the freedom and support for this natural process. It is important for us all, whether we are a parent, teacher, or friend to HSC's that we understand that the world will not change just because they want it to. They may have many problems in their lives throughout their life if they do not succeed in finding ways to deal with that sensitivity. We also need to provide them with ways of coping with those problems and help them find solutions so that they can live full, happy lives.

Although there are no specific treatments for HSCs other than psychological counseling, brief sessions of hypnotherapy seem to be helpful in reducing excessive inhibition and generalizing acquired confidence into everyday situations. There are no controlled studies, but some reports of the results from family therapy sessions suggest that these techniques seem to be helpful. Regular feedback on their performance is also a valuable way to reinforce their sense of effectiveness. It is important for HSC's to learn relaxation techniques and to breathe exercises since they can become upset by things that are not stressful, such as being called on in class or being told "no" by a teacher. The following websites provide additional information on dealing with highly sensitive children:

Several different theories have been proposed as potential causes of the sensitivity trait. These include the following: The "hard-wired" nature theory posits that sensory hypersensitivity has a strong genetic component, which is not in itself pathological but creates a vulnerability to environmental stressors. Thus, certain environmental events (such as trauma) may trigger the trait in genetically susceptible individuals. The "emotional regulation" or "arousal threshold" theories propose that oversensitivity is a result of problems in the modulation of arousal levels. Arousal is increased during periods of chronic stress; this internal dysregulation may manifest as behavioral and emotional problems or sensitization to external stimuli, such as smell and taste. The "sensitization" (often called "hyperresponsiveness" or "over-arousal") theory proposes that hypersensitivity has a biological basis and is a result of previous stimulation of the nervous system. Virtually all inputs become magnified and often result in intense activation of the perceiving system. Sensitivity may continue to increase after the stimulus is removed due to neuronal plasticity processes.

There are several models that try to explain HSC's, but they generally start with people who are in dire need of an explanation. In other words, they don't have one specific reason why HSC's are what they are, but they create an overall theory from assorted pieces of information.

The Neuroticism (sometimes called Emotional Stability) trait is a dimension of personality that encompasses such characteristics as anxiety, fearfulness, moodiness, irritability, and sensitivity. Neurotic people find it difficult to cope with stress, and they go to great lengths to avoid threats to their psychological well-being. The Conscientiousness trait reflects the extent to which a person is organized and hard-working. Conscientious people plan ahead and try to follow through on their intentions. They are generally seen as reliable and trustworthy. Those low in conscientiousness tend to be messy and disorganized or impulsive. They are often careless with money or procrastinate in completing tasks that they find unpleasant (such as paying bills).

The Achievement Orientation trait is a dimension of personality that includes such characteristics as self-confidence, motivation, and persistence. Those high in achievement orientation tend to be optimistic and believe that good things will happen to them and they can achieve their goals. They are often seen as hardworking, conscientious, bright, and energetic. Obsessive-Compulsive Personality Disorder is a mental illness characterized by repetitive behavior patterns that include preoccupation with orderliness and perfectionism. The disorder usually has a history of severe stress or trauma in the form of severe parental punitive behavior or other serious experiences which are emotionally distressing to the individual. Those individuals who suffer from this disorder are extremely fearful of making mistakes and tend to be over-conscientious, rigid, and extremely dedicated to work that often borders on perfectionism. There is no known cure for the genetic trait, but certain therapies can help in learning how to cope with the sensitivity factors. It is very important for adults who work with children that they understand how the hypersensitive child perceives and processes information and then find ways to cope with it. The following therapy methods have been found to be particularly successful:

Many highly sensitive children (HSC) have not had any problems through middle school or high school and may even excel in their academic lives by doing well on tests without studying much. However, as they work to get into university and college, they often find themselves in a very different academic world with much larger numbers of other students who have left classes early or come back to their academic lives with no intention of doing the required amount of study. Many HSCs who have been successful in middle school will find themselves struggling academically by the time they get to high school.

HSP's are especially vulnerable during high school when it comes to feeling negative emotions such as anger or fear from their peers because those feelings are particularly easily triggered by external events (such as comments from others). This can result in them getting overwhelmed if these feelings overpower their control mechanisms for dealing with the emotional intensity. Therefore, high school is a particularly difficult time for an HSC. It is important that parents and teachers understand that the typical high school years (between ages 13–17) are a particularly stressful time for this group because of their sensitivity and frequent reactions to the emotional intensity that are commonly experienced by those age groups.

There are many different factors that can cause an HSC to become unhappy in his or her academic life. One of the most common problems is feeling like no one understands what they're going through and being misunderstood by their teachers, parents, and other adults they come into contact with during school. They may feel misunderstood by their peers because the others don't understand what they are going through and may think that they are "weird" for having such strong feelings about things. The academic world is very different from the environment in which they were successful in middle school, so many of the fears and anxieties that they had to deal with then do not apply in a high school setting. HSCs need to learn how to cope with their emotions better, help them develop social skills, and find ways in which to fit into the more structured learning situation of high school. They also need to find ways to motivate themselves to study since many of them will require some extra help in doing so. Another issue that highly sensitive children often have is that they are very aware of how their peers react to them and often take those reactions personally. If they feel ignored by others or judged, they may react by getting angry at the person who has judged them (usually without any apparent reason). This type of response may be seen as "being too sensitive" and can lead to difficulties with peers. Again, this reaction could be due to a misunderstanding on the part of other students about the nature of HSCs' sensitivity. The following are a few things that HSC's can do to cope with negative emotions while they are in school:

- Homeschooling is becoming more popular in the United States, although not all highly sensitive children are advised to do so. Some parents believe that by sending their children away from the greater amount of external stimuli, they will be able to help them cope better. However, many students who have been highly sensitive find it difficult to adapt and may need special help while at home school. There is no problem for those who want to and feel ready for it, but many find their high sensitivity and emotional over-reactions make life at home difficult. Most parents have a hard time understanding how to help their HSC. This is especially difficult because they are typically described as "sensitive," and their reactions to the world may appear strange to the average person because of all of the conflicting emotions that they are experiencing. Their parents often ask, "Why can't he or she just deal with it?" It is important for parents to become educated about the evolution of their children's developing sensitivity and learn how to cope with it so that they can be more effective as co-admins.

- Highly sensitive children usually do well in elementary school but begin to struggle in middle school and high school since those years are usually extremely stressful for many teenagers, including HSCs. This can lead to a much more difficult time for those who are highly sensitive. It is important that they learn how to cope with their feelings and emotions more effectively since they often have trouble regulating them. It is also important that they learn to adjust the emotions they are expressing so they don't become overwhelmed by the intensity of the negative emotions that the world presents to them. They often find themselves without an adult role model in middle school and high school. This can make it hard for them to form friendships and sometimes even keep a positive attitude about themselves, especially when compared with their peers. Those who are able to discover the emotional intensity of their lives and are able to regulate their emotions better usually do well academically. There are a great many things that parents can do to support their HSCs in school. Some of these actions include:

Highly sensitive children sometimes face difficulties in reaching adulthood, specifically in the areas of working with other people and learning new skills. These difficulties can be due to being too sensitive or not having enough practice dealing with new situations with other people. Many people with HSCs do not have the confidence that their sensitivity is a normal part of life. They may be anxious and frightened about leaving home for the first time and may have little self-confidence in their new work environment. Learning how to cope with these feelings is the key to success despite the difficulties of living with this trait.

While most HSCs reach adulthood and embrace their high sensitivity, it does not mean that they should be considered pathological or weak. It just means that they are different from everyone else, which can sometimes make everyday challenges more difficult for them, but nothing they cannot learn and conquer. The following are some helpful methods for dealing with high sensitivity while in the workforce: There are many different therapies that have been developed to help HSCs cope with living life as adults. These often serve as supplements to the many other ways in which they take care of themselves. It is very important for HSCs to be guided through this important time period and be given support in their lives so that they can grow into healthy, happy adults.

Each year, thousands of children and teenagers die from hitting a wall of stress after going through a difficult transition where their previous environment has changed in some way, and they are experiencing more intense emotions than usual or are experiencing a loss or change of some kind (e.g., death of another family member or friend; divorce; loss of a friendship; and other such events). Some would define these deaths as suicide, but for various reasons (e.g., death due to driving into a wall while texting), most are deemed "accidents." Throughout the years, there have been many studies trying to find the correlation between highly sensitive people and suicide. Researchers found a connection between the two suggesting that highly sensitive people are at an increased risk of suicide. In addition, it was also noted that highly sensitive men were more likely to commit suicide than highly sensitive women, who may be linked with men not wanting to be seen as weak by killing themselves. In some cases, when a person is described as "too sensitive," what they usually are referring to is the hypersensitivity of the nervous system. Some people are born with a nervous system that is much more sensitive than others and thus find it difficult to cope with various aspects of daily living. Those who are born with hypersensitive nervous systems often have many more neurological sensitivities than other people because their nervous systems are too sensitive for them to cope effectively with certain environmental stimuli in ways that most people can. Common environmental stimuli include (but aren't limited to) lights, sounds, smells, and pain.

CHAPTER 15:

Personal Story

Monica was a Sensitive Child, and her family hoped that by giving her one-to-one attention, they would increase her self-confidence and develop her capabilities. But a Sensitive Child isn't necessarily a "special child," as the family soon found out.

She didn't seem to fit in with any of the other kids at the school. She was very bright, but her schoolwork was messy, her handwriting was poor, and she was too easily distracted by noises and people around her. She was often found staring into space, daydreaming. She was also a very friendly, loving, and caring child but at the same time quite needy, appearing to want constant affirmations. She seemed to have a hard time meeting the needs of her peers. I myself, more than once, had to threaten her with restrictions—she would have none of that, having been a very clever child.

Our Sensitive Child started experiencing emotional problems as early as four years old. About the same time, she developed a habit of staring into space for extended periods of time. Her grades started to drop, and her parents found her behavior very difficult to handle, particularly during meal times. Sometimes, she would suddenly get very sad and frightened and start crying. These episodes usually happened when she was in the presence of strangers or in a situation she found stressful.

When Monica was seven years old, her mother took her to see a child psychologist. The psychologist diagnosed Monica as being a Sensitive Child and recommended some exercises that would help her slow down some of the anxious over-response of other people. The exercises worked very well. After just a few months of practicing the Slow Down exercises, Monica became more confident and realized that she had a very high level of sensitivity and that her family could not respond to her needs perfectly all the time. She felt more comfortable with her responses. At the same time, her emotions started to lower, her concentration improved, and her relationships with her family and friends became more harmonious. She also learned to trust herself more and realized that she was very capable of taking care of her own needs.

At the age of eight, Monica told her mother that she was indeed a Sensitive Child and asked her if they could quit the "sensitizing treatments." When I met Monica, about a year later, she had been cured of all her sensitivity for at least a year. She was no longer a Sensitive Child. I worked with her for about a year before she began to respond to sensitizing sounds and pictures, but she had no sensitization to touch or pain. Severe sensitization usually develops sooner in Sensitive Children. We worked together for a couple of weeks before she fully regained her sensitization. After about fourteen months, her over-response had returned to normal.

Today, Monica is a very comfortable and happy adult. She has been married for three years and has a baby. She has been successfully employed in a full-time position. She is very successful and frequently travels. She bought her first house and still owns it today. She has plans for additional homes and knows how to handle money. She has returned to school and is receiving a degree in nursing. She is planning to become a nurse practitioner. It is my pleasure to know her.

Conclusion

Raising a highly sensitive child involves many new challenges, but one of the most common questions new parents ask is, "How can I make my childless sensitive?" This is a difficult task for any parent. An individual with high sensitivity will likely feel overwhelmed by loud noises, strong smells, and chaotic environments. If your child exhibits these tendencies to any degree, it's not so much that they need to be encouraged to become less sensitive as they need tools to manage their emotions and sensory reactions in order to function well in day-to-day life. Many parents try to change their child's sensitivity by using sensory integration therapy (SIT), which attempts to reduce the child's heightened reactivity to his or her environment. The general theory behind SIT is that children must learn to adapt to their surroundings, and that can only happen through repeated exposure—or "flooding"—with environmental triggers. But it's important for parents to understand the strong emotions a sensitive child feels when exposed to sensory inputs. For example, a powerful smell will often trigger intense emotional reactions, much like an intense stimulus would. The child may experience intense anger, sadness, fear, or even disgust. A child's emotions aren't always based on real events; some of the feelings may be more an attempt to cope with his or her environment than an event one is actually experiencing. Lacking the ability to control one's body's reaction to a situation can be very difficult for a highly sensitive child. He or she may be able to filter out certain noises or smells at home, but at school, they may become overwhelmed and cry because a loud noise made them dizzy. SIT seeks to desensitize children to specific stimuli through gradual exposure to them in order for the child's physical response to decreasing. Sensory stimuli will be used in conjunction with prompts such as clapping or tapping, which can help the child learn how to manage their emotional reactions. Combining SIT with biodynamic therapy (otherwise known as "biodynamic" or "bio-therapy") further helps by introducing growth factors into a child's environment. These growth factors are based on the same principles of bioregulation used in homeopathy; they're meant to help balance out a sensitive child's bodily reactions. Growth factors may be introduced into the home through a nursery or during homeopathic treatments for children, but they are also one of the ingredients used in some commercial products (such as "bioregenex"). Other, more common approaches to treating a child's sensitivity include counseling or educational methods. There are a number of books that have been written on this topic, such as the Gentle birth Guide series from Gentle Therapy for Children by Julia Gold and Heidi Ervin. The idea is that in order to treat a child's sensitivity, it is necessary to help parents learn about the issues directly related to their infant or child. Some parents may feel they deserve credit for having a sensitive child if they've encouraged their children to read using strategies like "stacking" books next to each other rather than tossing them aside occasionally. Other parents may be well aware that they have a sensitive child despite their best efforts to encourage him or her to fit in with the rest of the family. Parents with a highly sensitive child are sometimes surprised to find that their children are also often highly empathetic. Their strong sense of empathy usually stems from frustration at not being able to control their emotions and body's reactions, which can sometimes surface as intense anger, sadness, or fear. By teaching their children how to manage emotional reactions and helping them focus on positive ways they can help others (such as raising money for charity), parents can help their children become more confident in areas that aren't always easy for them. There are some children who are sensitive due to the presence of particular sensitivities, such as allergies. These children may be very prone to allergies due to stress due to their sensitivities, and living with them can be frustrating and upsetting for parents. However, many sensitive children also have allergies, and these may not be so severe that they impact their daily lives. Children with high sensitivity tend to have more anxiety in life than most other children do. They may possess a strong desire for independence and athletic abilities that other kids don't have. These traits may make them popular with other children, but that popularity can also create pressure to change things in order to fit in. A highly sensitive child may struggle with mental health issues due to the challenges of living with a highly reactive nervous system. They may have trouble sleeping and eat too little, which can increase feelings of anxiety and depression over time. Parents who are highly sensitive themselves naturally want to protect their children from every possible danger they can imagine; this desire for protection is based on concern for their child's safety and well-being. But not all parents who are sensitive have children that share those same sensitivities; this complicates matters when it comes to dealing with the child's overprotective tendencies. Many parents with highly sensitive children simply aren't aware that their children are highly sensitive due to their own lack of awareness. Some may feel that being sensitive is bad because it makes them feel different from others. But as more parents learn about the power of the brain and how it reacts to stimuli, they can help their children better understand themselves and manage their responses in a healthy way.

Dealing with overprotectiveness can be difficult for parents, especially in moments when they're feeling overwhelmed. They may not even realize they're overprotective until their children become frustrated and upset with them. It's best to help the child develop some coping mechanisms and to work toward desensitization so that your child can learn how to manage these emotions on his or her own. Parents of children who are extremely sensitive may also struggle with issues of their own, such as depression or anxiety, due to the challenges of parenting a sensitive child. It's important to understand your own reactions and emotions in order to deal with your children in an appropriate way. Tell them you love them and that you want them to be happy, even if they're not able to fit into those identifying with the mainstream. According to studies from New York University Professor Elaine Aron, the most sensitive adults share several characteristics that are present during childhood, including:

- Children who are extremely sensitive tend to have a higher level of empathy for others than average children do.
- They can often feel like they know how other people feel because they spend so much time observing others and considering how they might react under different circumstances.
- They often feel like they're being watched all the time, and they may believe that their family members are always judging them. This may lead to low self-esteem and feelings of stress or sadness if they are overprotected.
- A highly sensitive person is an individual who is easily overwhelmed by a normal level of stimulation, requiring more

than average to maintain an appropriate level of activity. This can cause them to have difficulty going about daily activities like eating, sleeping, and socializing. On the contrary, the less sensitive individual adapts quickly and easily to the amount of stimulus present in his surroundings.

- The highly sensitive person is often a perfectionist and may struggle to adjust to new or different situations. They may find their usual routines so stressful that they become physically ill when switching to new ones.
- The highly sensitive person can experience deep emotions due to their heightened sensitivity, including anger, sadness, anxiety, and stress which can lead to health problems like headaches, stomach ulcers, or depression.
- They are often good listeners who like to help others, but because they are constantly overstimulated by other people's feelings, they may make plans to avoid spending too much time with them. The highly sensitive person can be overwhelmed by the emotions or feelings of others and will need a quiet and calming environment away from crowds, loud noises, and lots of activity.
- The highly sensitive person can overanalyze the interactions with others and will want to be approved of by those around them. They may have a fear of failure leading to anxiety and depression.
- The highly sensitive person can become easily distracted, focusing on one thing at a time instead of everything happening at once. This often leaves them feeling overwhelmed and frustrated when other things take up their attention. They will often feel that they are neglecting their current tasks in favor of another task they have been planning to do.
- They can feel very anxious about the future because they are worried about what could happen next or how well they will cope with a change in circumstances or environment. A highly sensitive person can struggle with handling criticism. When they are the recipient of such feedback, they may become very upset and react in a way that does not reflect well on them.

They may feel that being mean or critical of them is justified because they have been treated in a mean way.

- HSP can be easily overwhelmed and can become frustrated when other people do not respond to their needs quickly enough and with the needed sensitivity.
- They can have difficulty standing up for themselves because they believe it will make them seem less worthy than others. This self-doubt about their personal worth can manifest as low self-esteem and feel like an outsider at times.
- They can feel overwhelmed by stimuli, which can cause them to become angry or upset and may experience feelings of discomfort and stress. They may become overwhelmed if they are not able to control the stimuli they are faced with.
- They feel emotional pain when something bad happens to someone they care about or someone they identify with. They will often feel extra emotional pain if they believe their loved one has been treated unfairly or mistreated.

The "highly sensitive person" (HSP) is not a real disorder (although the theory was developed by Elaine Aron, Ph.D., LISW, one of the founders of the field of empathy research). Dr. Aron's assertion that the HSP is a "situational disorder" is actually in contradiction to the Diagnostic and Statistical Manual of Mental Disorders (DSM-IV-TR) criteria for a number of diagnoses (e.g., anxiety disorders, personality disorders, and specific phobias). Furthermore, the DSM-5 has added an additional criterion for Major Depressive Disorder or Dysthymia: "OR... unexplained sensitivity/over-reactivity to environmental stimuli."

Sensitivity to environmental stimuli is not considered a "disorder" by mainstream medicine. In fact, as Dr. Aron stated in her paper: "For more than two decades, clinicians have been treating these children as if they had a “disorder,” but are now finally recognizing that there is nothing psychiatrically wrong with them. “In addition, the National Institutes of Health states that "Sensitivity to environmental stimuli runs along a spectrum. Some individuals may be just a little sensitive and may find it difficult to tune out loud sounds or strong odors. However, others may have unusual sensitivities, such as faint smells or tastes, which are overwhelming. “There is significant controversy over the use of the term "highly sensitive person" as well. Critics of Dr. Aron's theory state that "to the extent that being highly sensitive is a genetic trait, it is a genotype (not a personality characteristic) and thus isn't something a person has control over." Therefore, they argue, the term "highly sensitive person" implies weaknesses or deficits in an individual who is simply not true and could cause additional stress to people who may believe they have this innate tendency. Other critics argue that Dr. Aron's data may be accurate as to her individual research subjects; however, she has not demonstrated that her distinctions are valid or useful across different population groups or cultures. Her data have not been replicated by other researchers.

www.ingramcontent.com/pod-product-compliance
Ingram Content Group UK Ltd.
Pitfield, Milton Keynes, MK11 3LW, UK
UKHW021917190726
13853UKWH00002B/719